Your Birth Plan

A Step by Step Guide to Creating and Writing Your Birth Plan

Vanessa J. Merten

Pregnancy Podcast
864 Grand Avenue #543
San Diego, California 92109

www.PregnancyPodcast.com

ISBN: 978-1535586993
ISBN: 1535586990

First Edition.

The contents of this book ("Content") are for informational and educational purposes only. The Content is not intended to be a substitute for professional medical advice, diagnosis, or treatment. Always seek the advice of your physician, midwife, pediatrician, or other qualified health provider with any questions you may have regarding a medical condition. The Content is general in nature, and not specific to you, the reader, and is not intended as individual medical advice. The Content provided is intended as a sharing of knowledge and information and the author encourages you to make your own prenatal, birth, and postnatal care decisions based upon your research and in partnership with a qualified healthcare professional.

Table of Contents

Part One: The Basics of a Birth Plan

Chapter 1: Your Birth Plan

Your birth plan is the blueprint of how you envision your birth and what happens directly following the arrival of your baby. Once your birth plan is written this one piece of paper is going to have an abbreviated version of what is important to you, what you want to happen, and what you want to avoid.

A birth plan is really more than a piece of paper you give your care provider. A birth plan is the process you go through to prepare for the birth experience you want. The process of creating your birth plan is going to lay the foundation for you to be prepared for the scenario in which everything goes exactly as planned, and more importantly, for what should happen in the event things do not go as planned. The importance of a birth plan has a lot more to do with the process of writing it than it does with the finished product.

By the time you are finished with this book you are going to be really educated about everything that can impact your labor and birth. You will be on the same page as your care provider, your partner, and anyone else who will be by your side when you give birth. You are going to be confident in the decisions that you are making, and confident in your ability to have the birth experience you want. You will also be prepared for whatever happens on the magical day you get to meet your baby – even if things do not go as you envision. The more preparation that goes into your birth plan, the more you can be in control of your experience and the way in which your baby enters the world.

There are an infinite number of options you have as to how you plan your birth, and you always have options. Even if you end up having an emergency cesarean section, the planning you do during your pregnancy is going get you and your care provider prepared to handle things like what procedures are done with your baby as soon as they are born.

It is up to you whether you want to take ownership of choosing how your birth goes or if you want to leave all the decision making up to your doctor or midwife. If you are reading this book you are already on your way to having an empowered birth and setting yourself up for success to have the birth you want for yourself and your baby.

Chapter 2: Why You Need a Birth Plan

"If you fail to plan you plan to fail." – Benjamin Franklin

Going into labor without a plan is like running a marathon without any training or a roadmap of your route. The key to getting the birth you want is to plan. There are so many factors that are going to influence how your labor progresses, what procedures are done, and how your birth experience plays out. Your knowledge of these procedures and factors, and how you prepare for them, is going to determine what type of birth you have and how your baby enters the world.

If this is your first baby you are probably pretty overwhelmed with how much information is out there. Even if this is your second or third baby, each pregnancy and birth is so unique that there will always be unknowns. There are a lot of things that happen in between you going into labor until you are holding your beautiful new baby. Knowing what step is coming next, and how you want to handle it is going to prepare you to know what to expect.

You have options with infinite choices to make about everything during your pregnancy and birth. Your choices start with how you take care of yourself during your pregnancy, who you choose as your care provider, and what resources you trust for information. Your education will be the basis for you to find out what your options are. As you are creating your birth plan, you are going to find out your options and how your choices are going to affect you and your baby. Everything during labor is connected and understanding how one option will affect the next one is going to give you more control of the route you take to meeting your baby.

A birth plan allows you to make choices. You get to choose where you want to have your baby, who you want to be there, what procedures are done to you, and what procedures are done to your baby. If you don't make these choices someone else will make them for you. You know your body, your lifestyle, your preferences, and your priorities better than anyone. Would you plan a wedding by hiring a wedding planner, telling them to just take care of everything, make all of the decisions, and then plan to show up on your big wedding day and hope for the best? Planning a wedding is often a yearlong process of hashing out details to ensure everything goes just the way you want it. The day you give birth is one of the most important and amazing days of your life. The moment your baby is born will forever change who you are. Wouldn't you want to put the same care you would in planning for a wedding into making sure the very first day of your baby's life goes the way you want? How your day goes, and how you and your baby experience it is a direct result of your available options and choosing which options are best for you and your baby.

Chapter 3: Planning for the Unexpected

Labor is a bit of a wild card. There are so many variables and it can be tough to predict exactly how everything is going to go down on the big day. If you are a first-time mom having a baby is uncharted territory and there are a lot of unknowns. As you plan you have to be preparing for some flexibility. The more educated you are the better prepared you will be for whatever comes up.

Of course you are planning for the labor and birth experience you want but a big part of that is to know how will handle any situation. If you only plan for the best-case scenario and something unexpected happens suddenly you aren't in control.

Until you are in labor, there are a lot of things you will not know. Depending on the type of birth you are planning for, you have no idea when you will go into labor, or how long you will be in labor. You won't know whether any complications will come up, how you will cope with contractions, or how you will react to medications. You also will not know how your baby will handle labor and birth, or whether an emergency will come up. The unknown can be scary, but it doesn't have to be. You are on your way to being prepared for everything so you are going into your birth with confidence instead of uncertainty.

By preparing for anything you are setting yourself up for the best possible scenario no matter what happens. Knowing your plan B, understanding what you can do to avoid anything you do not want to be a part of your birth, and preparing for several scenarios is going to give you a better likelihood of everything going right.

Chapter 4: Building Your Team

Your Partner

Your partner's involvement starts with them going with you to your doctor or midwife appointments. You can expect to have somewhere around 14 appointments throughout your entire pregnancy. So on 14 days you will see a doctor or a midwife, that's it. Make it a priority for both of you to go to all of them, or at least attend as many together as you can. This gives your partner a chance to be included and have some input in any major medical decisions, ask any questions, and hear everything first hand.

Your partner needs to be involved in creating your birth plan and by the time it is done they should know it inside and out. They are going to be an advocate for you during your labor and birth. If they know exactly what your preferences are they will be able to speak up for you and help you get the birth experience you want.

Birth is one of the most physically and emotionally challenging workouts you will ever go through. Your partner won't just be sitting back and relaxing while this is going on. Your partner should expect to be there for you both physically and emotionally. Partners are a HUGE part of the birth of your baby. They are the cheerleader, coach, trainer, and major support. They need to be rested and prepared to be present for the entire thing. Your partner may also need to be an advocate for you and speak up in the event you are having trouble doing it. They should know what procedures you are on board with and what you want to avoid. Creating a birth plan is a great exercise for you two to get on the same page and get clear about what you do and do not want.

For more information for dads and partners you can listen to episode 13 of the Pregnancy Podcast at PregnancyPodcast.com/episode13.

Doula

A doula is a professional who has been trained in childbirth and who provides emotional, physical, and educational support to a mother and their birth partner. They are there to help with your labor, birth, and into the postpartum period. There are several types of doulas and a birth doula is someone you may want to consider involving in your birth experience. A birth doula usually meets up with you in your third trimester and helps you discuss and work through any anxiety and fears you have, will assist you in creating your birth plan, provide continuous support during your birth, and will provide nonjudgmental unbiased support to help you create the birth you want. Your doula doesn't just support you during your birth; they are also there to support your partner. Their expertise and experience with birth can be a huge advantage in helping your partner be right by your side and focused on you. A doula does not perform any medical procedures, deliver your baby, or give you any medical advice.

Having a doula attend your birth can be an amazing help in creating the birth experience you want. A doula can assist you whether you are having your baby at home or in a hospital setting, and whether you are planning a natural birth, or having a planned C-section. In a review of numerous studies, involving over 15,000 women, it was found that having continuous support during birth had a major impact on birth outcomes. Involving a doula will increase the likelihood of you having a spontaneous vaginal birth, meaning you wouldn't require any intervention to go into labor, decreases the likelihood of using pain medications if that is something you are wanting to avoid, decreases your risk of a C-section or an instrumental delivery with forceps or a vacuum, and decreases the length of your labor (Hodnett E.D., 2012).

For more information on doulas you can listen to episode 23 of the Pregnancy Podcast at PregnancyPodcast.com/episode23.

Choosing Your Care Provider

Choosing your care provider is the cornerstone of your prenatal care and birth experience. This is your expert resource that you will be working with throughout your pregnancy to make some very important decisions. You need to see them as an integral member of your team, and most importantly you need to trust them and be comfortable with them. Trust and confidence are as important as their qualifications, where they went to school, and how many babies they have delivered. It is absolutely critical that you include your care provider in discussions as you are creating your birth plan and that you work with them to come up with your plan. Creating a birth plan without their involvement is useless; they must be involved and supportive of your choices.

Generally, your primary care provider will be a midwife or an OB-GYN. Both types of professionals have to apply for a license, take an exam, and are required to complete continuing education throughout their career.

An OB-GYN is a doctor, but more specifically, they are an obstetrician/gynecologist. Obstetrics deals with pregnancy, childbirth, and the postpartum period, with a focus on situations requiring surgical interventions. Gynecology is focused on the health of the reproductive system and breasts. If you are in a high-risk pregnancy chances are you will be seeing an OB-GYN or a specialist. If you know you are planning a cesarean section you will be seeing an OB-GYN.

Midwives deal with pregnancy, childbirth, postpartum care and overall care for women. Midwives are not trained or licensed for surgery. Midwives specialize in normal, low-risk childbirth. Typically this means you don't have any complications. There are also Certified Nurse Midwives who are also Registered Nurses. If you are under the care of a midwife and something comes up which makes you high-risk, your midwife may get an OB-GYN involved, or if it is more appropriate, refer you to an OB-GYN for your care. Remember, most pregnancies are normal, low-risk, and require very little, if any, intervention.

Certified Nurse Midwives, Certified Midwives, or Professional Midwives, typically staff birth centers. A Certified Nurse Midwife has a bachelor's degree in nursing, and then goes through a 2-3 year graduate level training in midwifery. Certified Nurse Midwives are licensed in all 50 states in the U.S. Another credential is a Certified Midwife which does not have a nursing background, and Certified Midwives are only licensed in 5 states in the U.S. Certified Professional Midwives do not have college degree requirements, and instead gain their training through clinical training under the supervision of a midwife, and are only licensed in 27 states.

Both Midwives and OB-GYNs are highly regulated and go through a lot of education and experience before being licensed. They are different and each has its specialty.

Choosing your care provider isn't as black and white as having a baby at home with a midwife or having your baby at a hospital with an OB-GYN. The only way to know whether a particular person is the right fit for the pregnancy and birth you want is to ask questions and explore your options. Ultimately, your care provider will have a big impact on your experience and how your baby enters the world, and it is critical that you are on the same page and working towards the same goals.

There are some specific questions you can ask an OB-GYN or midwife when you are finding the right care provider.
What is your general philosophy on pregnancy care, labor, and birth?
How long have you been in practice?
How many births have you attended?
How many patients do you have at a given time?
Is your practice a solo or group practice? If it is a solo practice, who covers for you when you are not available?
How much time is available during each prenatal visit?
Are you available to answer questions in between visits?
Will you assist me to develop a birth plan or will you review one I have written?
What procedures are routine?
Will you be present throughout my labor?
Will you attend my birth? If you are unavailable, who will attend?

Questions if you are looking to avoid certain interventions:
What percentage of your patients utilize pain medication during labor?
What percentage of your patients has an episiotomy?
What is your C-section rate?

If you are interviewing a midwife you may also want to ask:
Did you graduate from a nationally accredited midwifery education program?
Are you certified by the American College of Nurse-Midwives?
Do you have an OB-GYN that you work with in the event one is needed?

Your doctor or midwife is your trusted partner during your pregnancy and labor. They are there to guide you through the process and ensure that you and your baby are healthy. Throughout your pregnancy you should have an open line of communication with them about what you do and do not want during your labor and birth and it is critical that you are on the same page.

Your doctor or midwife has years of education, training, and experience and they will have policies, procedures, and opinions that will impact how things go on the big day. Communicating with your care provider about your birth plan involves knowing what their policies and procedures are so you can plan accordingly. You will be relying on their knowledge and expertise to guide you through a lot of decision-making. Including them in making your birth plan is critical to you getting the birth experience you want.

For more information on choosing the right care provider you can listen to episode 34 of the Pregnancy Podcast at PregnancyPodcast.com/episode34.

Additional People

If there is anyone else that you want by your side through your labor and birth you are welcome to include them in your planning. This could be a sibling, your mom, your favorite aunt, anyone you want. The decision to include anyone in your birth should be your decision. Do not let anyone pressure you into having him or her there if that is not what you want. If you do choose to have someone additional present, they don't necessarily need to be involved in making the decisions that go into your plan. However, you do want them to be clear on what your plan is, and what their role is.

Part Two: What to Include

Chapter 5: Planning for Your Venue

Where you choose to have your baby is going to have a lot of influence on the type of birth you are planning. Birth is not an all or nothing decision where you are either having a baby in hospital with tons of interventions, or having a baby at home with no interventions. There are an infinite number of options available to you to really prepare for and craft the birth experience you want. Whether you are planning to give birth at home, at a birth center, or in a hospital, each venue has its pros and cons. This chapter explores these three options and gets into some of the things you will want to take into consideration when planning your home, birth center, or hospital birth.

If you are planning to have your baby at home or in a birth center there is always the possibility you could end up at the hospital. You can have your birth plan for your home or birth center birth, and also create a plan B in the event you end up in the hospital. Hopefully it stays tucked away and you never have to use it, but it will give you some peace of mind that you are prepared for anything.

Hospital

Whether you are planning a cesarean section or having a natural labor you could do either in a hospital. About 98% of all births in the United States are in hospitals so if you live in the U.S. there is a good chance that is where you are planning to give birth.

It is likely that you have more than one hospital in your area. Use the selection to your advantage to shop around and find the hospital that is the best fit for you. A hospital will give you a tour, which will give you a good feel for the labor and delivery unit, the staff, and the overall environment. There could be big differences in how you feel at one hospital compared to another so shop around and go with the one you think will be the best fit for the birth experience you want.

It is really important to know what the policies of your doctor or midwife are, and what the policies of the hospital are. Hospitals are major organizations. They have policies and procedures in place to protect both patients and hospital staff. These policies will have an impact on your labor, birth, and stay. If there are any interventions you would like to include, or if there are any that you would like to avoid, talk to your care provider about what the policy of the hospital is beforehand so you can plan accordingly.

It is a good idea to talk to your doctor or midwife before you go into labor to find out if they will be there for your labor and birth, when during the process they will show up, and how long they will stay. In some cases you won't see your care provider until you are ready to push. You want to know what their policy is beforehand so you are not disappointed when you expect them to be there and they aren't. It is also possible that you have had your prenatal care at a practice with several doctors or midwives and the person who will be present for your birth is the person who happens to be on call when you go into labor. Generally you will have several nurses taking excellent care of you during most of your labor and they will alert your doctor or midwife when they need to be there. Talk to your care provider beforehand so you know when you can expect to see them.

A pro to being at a hospital is that they should be equipped for any type of emergency. You could be planning on having your baby in a hospital setting if you have a high-risk pregnancy or if your care provider is expecting any complications. Keep in mind that most births do not involve an emergency, but if this is something that you are concerned about you can rest assured that the hospital and staff are well equipped to handle anything.

There are many procedures and amenities that are only available at a hospital. This would include continuous electronic fetal monitoring, availability of an epidural or Pitocin, and the ability to have a cesarean section. All of these interventions and more are covered in depth in chapter 8.

When you are about to deliver, you will find that there are suddenly more people in your hospital room. In general there will be at least three nurses, and your OB-GYN or your midwife. Once your little one is born there will probably also be a pediatrician or a family physician there to check in on your baby, while your care provider is checking on you.

In most cases, your care provider will put your baby directly on your chest right after birth. If there are any issues of course they will address those, their number one job is to make sure you and your baby are healthy. The good news is that you are in a hospital so if anything isn't perfect they have the staff and the resources to treat it.

How long you stay at the hospital depends on several factors including the policy of the hospital, and how you and your little one are doing. Most moms spend 24-48 hours in the hospital. You may end up spending a longer amount of time there; it is really going to be on a case-by-case basis. Make sure you discuss the length of your stay with your care provider, well before you go into labor, so you know what the policy of the hospital is and what you can expect. Once you have your baby, if you are feeling ready to go home or maybe not quite ready to leave, speak up and find out what your options are. Chances are you will be spending at least one night in the hospital, and your partner can spend the night with you. Some hospitals or rooms will be equipped with a chair that turns into a bed or a cot for your partner. You can always ask your care provider what the accommodations are at the hospital and you can bring a pillow or anything else that would help your partner be more comfortable.

Take advantage of being surrounded by so many experts in the hospital. This is especially true after your baby arrives. You can get assistance with breastfeeding, swaddling, if you have questions about how to change a diaper, whether your baby's sleeping is normal, whatever questions you have, ask them. Take advantage of the staff while you have access to them. It is likely the hospital has a lactation consultant on site. Have them come by for a short visit. Getting off on the right foot with breastfeeding can make a huge difference for both you and your baby.

On the other hand you may find that you just need a little peace and quiet and some time without people constantly going in and out your room to check on you or your baby. Ask your nurse or care provider if you can get a few hours without being disturbed, or perhaps you can put a do not disturb sign on your door. It is not unreasonable to ask for a break from people coming in and out of your room at all hours to check on you or your baby.

Keep in mind you are the captain of the ship. It is up to you to make informed decisions and even if something is routine, you have options. Throughout your pregnancy you will be working with your care provider on your birth plan. Although you should see eye to eye on things by the time you go into labor do not hesitate to ask questions and remind them that you have a birth plan, and what your wishes are.

For more information on hospitals you can listen to episode 37 of the Pregnancy Podcast at PregnancyPodcast.com/episode37.

Home

It was not too long ago in our history that all births took place at home. Over the last century the number of women giving birth at home has sharply declined. The decline in home births is due to many factors beyond just the advancements we have made in medicine. The laws of your country or state, the coverage of home birth by your insurance or health care, and social attitudes have all played a part in directing where you go to have your baby.

Home births are natural births and almost always attended by a midwife. You will not have access to an epidural, continuous electronic fetal monitoring, or Pitocin. In the U.S. midwives cannot legally use forceps or a vacuum for an assisted delivery. A midwife can perform an episiotomy if necessary, although it is pretty rare. Overall, intervention use is much lower with midwife-led care than doctor led care. For many women the unavailability of these interventions is a big reason they choose home birth with a midwife and it is by design that most interventions are avoided in home births.

Home births are less expensive than hospital births, but they are not always covered by insurance. You will need to check with your care provider and your health coverage to find out if home birth is covered. It could also be a good idea to find out how your insurance coverage will work in the event you do end up at the hospital, just so you are prepared for anything. Trying to locate this information online may be tough and getting on the phone with your health insurance may be more helpful. You might be on a hold for a little bit before you will reach someone but in the long run you will save time and get direct answers to your specific questions.

Worldwide the most popular choice of place to have a baby is not at home. As of 2012 about .89% of all births in the United States took place at home. This was a pretty big increase from just .54% in 2004 (MacDorman M.F., 2014). As of 2013 in the U.K. 2.3% of births took place at home (Office for National Statistics, 2014). As of 2013 only .3% of births in Australia occurred at home (Australian Institute of Health and Welfare, 2013). In Canada public health coverage of home birth services varies from province to province, as does the availability of doctors and midwives providing home birth services. In Ontario about 2.49% of births were home births in 2013 (Murray-Davis B., 2015). In British Columbia just over 4% of births take place at home, and this is the highest rate of any province in Canada (Midwives Association of British Columbia, 2010).

If you are planning a home birth you will be working closely with your midwife to plan the details of your birth and it is really important to know what the policies of your midwife are. They will be knowledgeable on the governing laws where you live that could affect your birth. Most jurisdictions will have some type of criteria a woman needs to meet for a midwife to attend a home birth. An example of this could be that you need to give birth between 37 and 42 weeks.

In 23 U.S. states there are no licensing laws for direct-entry midwives or Certified Professional Midwives, and practicing midwives can be arrested for practicing medicine without a license (Midwives Alliance North America). If the state you live in does not have licensing for direct entry or Professional Midwives your only option for an attended home birth is with a Certified Nurse Midwife, since they are licensed in all 50 states.

If you and your midwife are planning for a home birth you two will be doing everything you can to support that. The number one priority of your midwife is the safety of you and your baby. Generally speaking, home births are low-risk pregnancies without complications. Throughout your prenatal care you will be monitored by your midwife who will be making sure everything is going smoothly, that you remain low-risk, and that home birth is still a good option for you. Prenatal visits could be at your home, the midwife's home, or at a clinic.

You will probably need some supplies for a home birth that you would not need if you were having a baby in a birth center or hospital. Ask your midwife what you need, they should be able to give you a list of supplies and let you know what they will be providing. There is a perception that home birth is really messy. It doesn't have to be and with some planning ahead of time cleanup is super easy. You will be bonding with your baby after birth so you do not need to worry about cleanup, that will be done by the midwife, your partner, and anyone else there to help. Some items you may want to consider are protective coverings for your floor and furniture. This could be plastic or rubber sheeting, a shower curtain, towels, sheets, or large disposable pads. You may want some type of protective covering for your bed. Some other items you may want to have on hand are a birthing ball or any other equipment or tools you plan to use during labor. A mirror so you can see your baby's head crown, if you think that may be helpful. Food and drinks for both during and after labor, for you, and anyone else who will be there, and anything else that would be helpful. Luckily you are at home, and everything you own is within reach. You may want to pack an emergency bag in case you need to transfer to a hospital. For more information on what to pack in your hospital or birth center bag you can listen to episode 24 of the Pregnancy podcast at PregnancyPodcast.com/episode24 and download a free checklist. You should have all the supplies on hand that you need by week 37, just in case your little boy or girl decides to show up early.

If you are considering a water birth there may be some additional supplies you need. You can read more on water birth in chapter 10.

At the start of your labor you are going to call your midwife. They may head over to your house right away and be involved right from the beginning of labor, or they may wait until your labor has progressed. You should discuss this with them beforehand so you know when you can expect them to come to your house. Home births frequently have several support people present like your partner, another family member, friend, or a doula. Your midwife will primarily be running point to let you do what you need to do during labor with your partner or doula, and of course if you need their support in any capacity they are there for that. They will be monitoring you and your baby and make sure everything is going smoothly. A home setting will give you a lot of freedom for how you labor in different places and positions. You will be able to eat or drink whatever you want. This is encouraged because you will be expending a lot of energy in labor and you will need fuel and to stay hydrated. You can have your partner or another family member catch your baby when they are born and when you meet that little boy or girl they will be placed skin to skin on your chest immediately. Your home environment will allow you to be in control of how and where you labor.

Once your baby is born your midwife will be checking you and your baby to make sure everyone is healthy and doing well. Especially in a home setting, you really get to enjoy the time after birth without interruption and focus on bonding. After delayed clamping, your midwife will be cutting the umbilical cord, unless your partner or someone else wants to do it. Once the placenta is out they will be disposing of that, unless you are keeping it for encapsulation. At some point they will also weigh and measure your baby but the focus is on allowing you to bond with your little one and they will work around that.

Since you are not in a hospital, you will be advised to take your baby to see a pediatrician within three days after birth. Have a pediatrician already picked out and make sure they know that you are planning a home birth, that they are supportive of that, and will get you an appointment right away after your baby is born.

The big question surrounding home birth is, is it safe? Following are some of the key studies so you can decide for yourself whether or not you feel home birth is a safe option.

Overall, studies show a lower rate of interventions in home births including epidural analgesia, electronic fetal heart rate monitoring, episiotomy, and operative vaginal and cesarean deliveries. Women who planned birth at home also had fewer infections, less perineal and vaginal lacerations, hemorrhages, and retained placentas. Home births compared to hospital births also are associated with a higher overall satisfaction with the experience from women who gave birth at home (International Journal of Women's Health, 2015).

The official statement of the American Congress of Obstetricians and Gynecologists (ACOG) is that although the Committee on Obstetric Practice believes that hospitals and birthing centers are the safest setting for birth, it respects the right of a woman to make a medically informed decision about delivery. Women inquiring about planned home birth should be informed of its risks and benefits based on recent evidence. Specifically, they should be informed that although the absolute risk may be low, planned home birth is associated with a twofold to threefold increased risk of neonatal death when compared with planned hospital birth. Importantly, women should be informed that the appropriate selection of candidates for home birth; the availability of a Certified Nurse Midwife, Certified Midwife, or physician practicing within an integrated and regulated health system; ready access to consultation; and assurance of safe and timely transport to nearby hospitals are critical to reducing perinatal mortality rates and achieving favorable home birth outcomes (American Congress of Obstetricians and Gynecologists, 2011).

The stats cited in the opinion of the American Congress for Obstetricians and Gynecologists comes from a meta-analysis by the American Journal of Obstetrics and Gynecology of 12 studies which included a total of over 340,000 planned home births and over 207,000 planned hospital births. A meta-analysis is an analysis that combines results of several studies. The big focus of this study is that the overall neonatal death rate was almost twice as high in planned home versus planned hospital births. There was no difference found in perinatal death for home versus hospital births. Neonatal death occurs within the first four weeks of life, whereas perinatal is within the first week, and includes stillborn babies. This study was a controversial one in the midwife community and there are some concerns raised about the methods and the data (Hart, 2010).

A review published by the International Journal of Women's Health in 2015 looked into 31 studies published primarily in the last 10 years from a lot of different countries. This review is not a meta-analysis, so data from multiple studies is not combined. The review concluded that while evidence regarding neonatal outcomes related to home birth remains inconclusive, what is clear is that when guidelines and systems of transfer are in place, there is either minimal or no increased risk associated with home birth for low-risk women (Zielinski R., 2015).

A study from the Netherlands, where home birth rates are among the highest in the world, found no increased risk of adverse perinatal outcomes for planned home births among low-risk women. This included over 743,000 women. The authors noted that the results might only apply to regions where home births are well integrated into the maternity care system (Jonge A., 2014).

Here is where the research gets even more confusing. The 2014 Netherlands study was an update of one originally done in 2009. The 2009 study included over 500,000 women and data from this was used in the results of the meta-analysis used by the American Journal of Obstetrics and Gynecology, however, data from the Netherlands study on neonatal mortality was excluded. The findings on the high rates of neonatal mortality were the basis of ACOG's argument against the safety of home birth, and had all of the results from the Netherlands study been included; the numbers would have been much lower (Jonge A., 2014).

If you are planning a home birth you should still have a solid backup plan. There is always the possibility you could be transferred to a hospital. Some reasons you could be transferred to a hospital are; if labor isn't progressing, if you have meconium in your amniotic fluid, a placental abruption, umbilical cord prolapse, if you do not deliver the placenta or it's not intact, or if your baby shows signs of distress, like an abnormal heart rate or trouble breathing. There is also the possibility that you decide you want to transfer to a hospital. A big part of planning a home birth is knowing what your plan is in the event things do not go as you envision. Most transfers to a hospital are not calls to an ambulance in a dire emergency. Often there are signs that a transfer would be beneficial way before an emergency arises. Some hospital transfers still result in a natural birth so don't assume that transferring automatically means you will be having an emergency C-section. Talk to your midwife about what happens if you want to go to a hospital. You should know to whom your care transfers to and whether your midwife would stay with you for your labor in the hospital. Most importantly, you need to know that whatever happens is okay. A planned home birth that ends up in a hospital is not a failure. Sometimes things do not go as planned, and that is okay.

For more information on home birth you can listen to episode 42 of the Pregnancy podcast at PregnancyPodcast.com/episode42.

Birth Center

A birth center is a middle ground between a home birth and a hospital. You get the benefit of a natural birth, with some of the safety net that you would have in a hospital setting. Birth centers are generally based on midwife-led care focused on prenatal and postpartum care for low-risk women. The majority of birth centers are freestanding centers completely separate from a hospital. More birth centers are popping up in hospitals with the same focus of natural birth but they are fully integrated within the hospital system in the event resources or care from the hospital are needed.

Birth Centers are becoming more popular in the U.S. In 2004 there were 170 birth centers and a total of .23% of births took place in a freestanding birth center. By 2013 there were 248 birth centers, which accounted for .39% of births. The number of women giving birth in a birth center is still less than home births but the number will continue to grow as more birth centers pop up around the country (MacDorman M.F., 2014).

The Commission for Accreditation of Birth Centers certifies birth centers that meet standards set by the American Association of Birth Centers.

Many birth centers will also work closely with other professionals like nurses, acupuncturists, doulas, massage therapists, counselors, chiropractors, childbirth educators, nutritionists, and lactation consultants. Some birth centers will have some of these professionals on staff, or have a close working relationship with professionals they can recommend and refer you to. Birth centers strive to be a comprehensive one-stop shop for your prenatal, birth, and postpartum care.

The cost of prenatal care and birth tends to be less expensive at a birth center compared to a hospital. You will need to check with the birth center and your health insurance to find out if a birth center is covered, and up to what amount. It could also be a good idea to find out how your insurance coverage will work in the event you do end up at the hospital, just so you are prepared for anything. Some birth centers may offer assistance or reduced rates if you are low-income. If you are concerned about the cost ask if there are any programs you could qualify for to reduce the fees.

If you have more than one birth center in your area go check them out and ask for a tour. This will give you an opportunity to meet some of the midwives and get a feel for the place to see if it would be the right fit for you. Birth centers are unique settings and there can be big differences between them. If you are looking at a couple options you may also want to find out the proximity to a hospital or the procedures in place at each center if a transfer becomes necessary. You also can, and should, have a tour of your backup hospital. If you have multiple hospitals in your area, go tour them so you can choose the best one for you in the event you end up there.

Birth centers focus on wellness care for low-risk women. Your prenatal appointments will take place at the birth center, they tend to be longer than typical appointments with an OB-GYN, and focus on education and answering any questions you have. Many birth centers will involve you as much as possible in your prenatal care from asking you to take some tests at home to checking your own weight. You are much more of an active participant, rather than a patient at a birth center. You being an active participant is part of the model of midwife-led care.

Depending on the structure of the birth center you may have an assigned midwife who will be present for your birth or you could end up with the midwife on call. Make sure you know the policy of the birth center so you know who you can expect to be present for your birth.

The labor and birth experience at a birth center is very similar to a home birth, both in the setting and the policies. In a birth center you are encouraged to eat and drink to keep your energy levels up. A birth center is set up like a home setting; there is usually a bed, tools like squatting bars and birthing balls, and often a tub for water births. Midwives in a birth center encourage you to labor in the way that is most beneficial for you, and however and wherever you are most comfortable.

Birth centers do not utilize or offer most interventions like routine IV fluids, continuous electronic fetal monitoring, inductions, epidurals, or assisted delivery. Generally for these interventions you would need to be transferred to a hospital. The rate of episiotomies tends to be really low at birth centers, but if one is needed your midwife can perform one. For more information on episiotomies and some things you can do to avoid tearing and an episiotomy you can listen to episode 22 of the Pregnancy podcast at PregnancyPodcast.com/episode22.

Birth centers should have procedures in place in the event a transfer to a hospital is needed. In most cases if you need to be transferred it is not an emergency situation. You should discuss how this works and whether your midwife would be able to continue your care in a hospital or whether they would transfer you to an OB-GYN. The birth center should have OB-GYNs they work with regularly and that are supportive of natural birth.

After the birth of your baby you can expect to be able to focus on your little one. Your midwife will of course be checking to make sure both you and baby are healthy and doing fine. Your stay after birth at a birth center is much shorter than a hospital stay and often you can expect to go home the same day. Talk to your midwife ahead of time so you know how long you can expect to be there.

Now that you have an overview of what a birth center is and how it works, let's examine some of the statistics and the safety concerns at birth centers. There is not a ton of research on birth centers, and as more open up around the country, hopefully we will see more published data. Keep in mind women who are good candidates for prenatal care and birth at a birth center are low-risk without complications.

A study of over 15,000 women who planned to give birth at birth centers between 2007 and 2010 has some great stats to give you a good idea of why some women choose to give birth at a birth center. 94% had a vaginal birth. This means that the C-section rate for low-risk women who chose to give birth at a birth center was only 6%, of course the women who had a cesarean were transferred to a hospital. 84% of women were able to give birth at the birth center. Of all of the participants, 4.5% were referred to a hospital before being admitted to the birth center, 11.9% transferred to the hospital during labor, 2.0% transferred after giving birth, and 2.2% had their babies transferred after birth. Of the women who transferred to a hospital during labor, 54% ended up with a vaginal birth, 8% had a forceps or vacuum-assisted vaginal birth, and 38% had a C-section. The majority of the in-labor transfers were for non-emergency reasons, such as prolonged labor. 0.9% of the total participants transferred to the hospital during labor for emergency reasons, 0.4% of mothers, and 0.6% of newborns transferred after birth for emergency reasons (Dekker, 2013).

For more information on birth centers you can listen to episode 44 of the Pregnancy Podcast at PregnancyPodcast.com/episode44.

Chapter 6: Labor Room Environment

In the wild most animals retreat to a quiet safe place to give birth. If there is any sign of danger their bodies will literally halt the birth so they can react to the threat and find safety. Humans operate the same way. Oxytocin is a major hormone during birth. It isn't a coincidence that this is also the hormone released when you have an orgasm. Oxytocin is known as the love hormone and many people argue that the environment you give birth in should be similar to the environment you make love in. Your labor will progress best in an environment where you feel safe and relaxed. No matter where you are having your baby you could make some adjustments to your surroundings to create the environment that works best for you.

Bright light is perfect for a beach day but may not be perfect for birth. Even in a hospital filled with fluorescent lighting you can shut off some of the lights or possibly dim them if you find it helpful. If your care provider or a nurse needs brighter lights for a specific procedure you can ask them to dim or turn off some of the lights when they are not needed. Candles may not be permitted at a birth center or hospital due to fire risk. An alternative would be to use battery powered candles. Some birth centers may have these available and if not you can always bring them with you.

Sound can be a game changer for your environment. This could include music, meditations, or even white noise or ocean sounds to drown out other noises that can be a distraction. Often you can request to turn the volume down or off on monitors or other machines that beep or make noises. Even the volume of voices can affect your environment. If you prefer to keep your labor room as quiet as possible do not hesitate to ask anyone present to speak at a low volume if that is important to you. When your baby is born they will be able to recognize your voice and your partners voice and the quieter the room is the better they will be able to hear you and know mama is right there.

Your sense of smell can have an impact on your mood and your environment. Essential oils are becoming increasingly popular for use in labor for relaxation. Diffusing oils may be against the policy of a hospital or birth center and it would be helpful to know what their policy is before bringing a diffuser with you. If you are interested in incorporating essential oils in your labor and birth it may be helpful to put oils on cotton balls and store them in a Ziploc bag. In the event a particular scent is no longer helpful for you, it is much easier to seal up a plastic bag and open a new one, than to clear the air and get a smell out of an entire room from a diffuser. Not all essential oils are recommended for expecting moms and if you have any concerns about using particular oils consult your care provider.

A great way to make any environment feel more like home is to add pictures. This could be a picture of your family, a drawing from a big brother or sister to be, or an affirmation that you want to be reminded of during your labor.

During your labor and birth you should be surrounded by supportive people you have invited to be in your space. If someone is there it should be because you asked him or her to be there. Do not let anyone pressure you into including him or her if you do not want them present. This is your day and you are running the show.

Someone you may want to include is a birth photographer to document your day. If this is something you are considering talk to the photographer beforehand about your labor room environment so they can plan ahead to work with the lighting and surroundings you prefer. If you want photos of the birth it is a good idea to coordinate with your care provider to find out what their guidelines are for photography.

Overall your labor environment needs to be a place that you feel comfortable in. If there is something that you could add to your space that would make a difference for you add it. If something about the environment is not working for you, ask if you can adjust it, remove it, or turn it off. The more comfortable you are in your surroundings the more relaxed and at ease you will be to focus on meeting your baby.

For more information on your labor room environment you can listen to episode 41 of the Pregnancy Podcast at PregnancyPodcast.com/episode41.

Chapter 7: Labor Positions

For most of our entire human history a mother in labor was free to move around and change positions to whatever was most comfortable and suited her best at the time. It really wasn't until we made labor and birth a medical process that women began laboring on their backs in a bed. There was even a time when the mom was strapped and restrained to a bed to make sure she stayed put. Can you believe that? Part of the changing of our practice, especially in the United States, was a shift of the focus from the birthing mother to the doctor delivering the baby. A mom on her back in a bed made the doctor's job much easier because they had access to see everything going on. Convenience for the doctor doesn't necessarily equate to the best position for the mother. Some of the negatives of lying on your back with your legs raised are that it works against gravity, your major blood vessels are compressed, and there is a higher probability of a vaginal tear or an episiotomy.

When you are in labor you may not be thinking 100% clearly, and may not recall all of the positions you prepared for during your pregnancy. This is an area where your partner can really come in handy. Go over positions with your partner so that when you are preoccupied with giving birth to your little one your partner can help to suggest some other positions. Also, if there are any positions they are physically supporting you in they will know what to do. If you are having a doula attend your birth they will also be an excellent resource of ideas of some different positions to try.

Standing and walking can be especially helpful in the early stages of labor. Standing and walking use gravity so it is going to encourage your baby to descend further into your pelvis. It helps deliver more oxygen to your little one, it may speed up labor, and it may make contractions more comfortable for you than if you were sitting or lying down. A walk is also a great distraction to spend some time in the earliest stage of labor. Walking may not be recommended if you have high blood pressure, and if you have any questions about that please bring them up with your care provider.

Especially during the first stage of labor, when your cervix is dilating and effacing, you really want to work with gravity, not against it. In a review of women during the first stage of labor, it was concluded that there is clear and important evidence that walking and upright positions in the first stage of labor reduces the duration of labor, the risk of cesarean birth, the need for epidural, and does not seem to be associated with increased intervention or negative effects on mothers' and babies' well-being. Better quality trials are still required to confirm with any confidence the true risks and benefits of upright and mobile positions compared with recumbent, or lying down, positions (Lawrence A., 2013).

Some positions you may find helpful in the earlier stages of labor are:
Rhythmic moving like swaying or rocking, if mobility is limited, even sitting in a rocking chair, if one is available, can be helpful
Lunging may be able to help your little one rotate, if they are not in the optimal position, and can help them descend
Sitting on a bed, chair, or toilet facing forward or backwards
Hands and knees or kneeling
Lying on your side, particularly lying on your left side, as that will maximize blood flow to your uterus and your baby

There are some props that may assist you during labor and this could include:
Birthing ball
Squatting bar
A bed sheet to knot and use over a door or to loop around a squatting bar to help pull you up and use as leverage
Birthing stool
If you want to utilize any of these during your labor or birth find out if they will be available where you are giving birth or if you need to bring them with you. If you are including a doula they may also be able to provide some tools or props for you.

Squatting in particular is really helpful for the second, or pushing stage. When you squat the opening of your pelvis increases, which gives your little one more room. Squatting encourages your baby to descend downwards better than any other position. In a squatting position you are still able to shift your weight around and maintain some movement. It is great for circulation of blood to your baby, it may increase their rotation, and overall squatting makes it easier for your little one to make their way out.

In one review that compared women who labored in the second stage of labor, researchers concluded that women should be allowed to make choices about the birth positions they might wish to assume. Overall the findings suggested several benefits to being in an upright position for women who did not have an epidural, but there was also an increased risk of blood loss. Specific to the benefits, the researchers found that for women who labored during the second stage in an upright position there was a 27% decrease in assisted deliveries, a 7% decrease in episiotomies, and fewer abnormal fetal heart rate patterns (Gupta J.K., 2012).

If you are limited in your mobility you still have options for positions. Even hooked up to an IV pole or a fetal monitor you will have some room to move, sit up, squat, or stand.

There was a study done in Italy that concluded women should be encouraged to move and deliver in the most comfortable position for them. This study compared women giving birth in an upright position to women who labored and gave birth lying down. Women who used upright positions more than 50% of the time had more effective uterine contractions and more perineal muscle relaxation, and their births were significantly shorter. In addition they had lower rates of request for epidurals or other medication, less assisted deliveries, and less cesarean sections. The study notes that no differences were found in terms of neonatal outcomes (Gizzo S., 2014).

You can see that there is definitely scientific evidence showing a benefit to being in an upright position. Overall the studies really show that you should have the freedom to move as you see fit. If you have any limitations due to interventions during your labor and birth, work with your care provider to find the best positions for those circumstances. If you are uncomfortable and want to try a different position, definitely speak up.

For more information on labor positions you can listen to episode 36 of the Pregnancy Podcast at PregnancyPodcast.com/episode36.

Chapter 8: Interventions

An intervention is any procedure performed by a care provider to assist in the delivery of your baby. Interventions include inductions, continuous electronic fetal monitoring, administering IV fluids, antibiotics for group B strep, an epidural, episiotomy, assisted delivery (using forceps or a vent house suction cup), and a cesarean. By learning what each procedure entails, and when and why it is performed, you will be better able to make decisions as to whether or not you really need or want to include it in your birth plan.

Modern medicine is amazing and there is no doubt that lives of both mothers and babies have been saved by interventions. When they are needed we are very lucky to have access to medical interventions. All interventions carry risks with them. Remember, your job is to make informed decisions based on what is best for you and your baby. Just because something is suggested by a care provider does not mean it is mandatory, and you always have the final say.

For any intervention there are some excellent questions you can ask your care provider before opting into a procedure:
Why do I need this procedure?
What are the benefits to my baby and me?
Are there other options available? If there are, what are they?
What are the risks of the procedure?
What are the risks if the procedure isn't done?
Can I delay the procedure? Wait an hour or a day and what are the risks of delaying the intervention?

For more information on interventions you can listen to episode 8 of the Pregnancy Podcast at PregnancyPodcast.com/episode8.

Induction

You already know that pregnancy is measured in 40 weeks and your due date is the end of week 40, or about 280 days from your last menstrual period. This calculation assumes a 28-day cycle, with ovulation about day 14. Your due date is an estimate of when your baby will arrive; it is not an exact science. Often when your baby is late, it is likely that they really aren't late at all, but rather, your due date is off.

Inducing labor is any procedure that is used to stimulate uterine contractions during pregnancy before labor begins on its own. A care provider may recommend inducing labor for various reasons and primarily an induction is recommended when there's concern for the health of mom or baby. Weighing the risks of an induction against the benefits will help you decide if this is the best course of action for you and your baby.

The last few weeks of pregnancy are really critical to your baby's development. Maternal antibodies are being passed to your baby—these will help fight infections in their first days and weeks of life. Your baby is gaining weight and strength, they are increasing iron stores, and developing more coordinated sucking and swallowing abilities. The last few weeks are also when your little one's lungs mature and prepare for that first breath of air. Your baby is storing brown fat that will help them maintain their body temperature in the first weeks following birth. As your baby and your body get ready to go into labor your placenta triggers an increase in prostaglandin that softens the cervix to prepare it for effacing and dilating. Your levels of estrogen rise, and the levels of progesterone decrease which makes the uterus more sensitive to oxytocin, which is the hormone responsible for contractions. Nearing labor your baby will move further down into the pelvis. While all of this is going on internally you may notice that you have extra energy, which allows you to make any final preparations, and you may have trouble sleeping, which is thought to help prepare you for being awake at all hours with a new baby. It is really this symphony of everything working together in sync that starts your labor. In a perfect world, everything works like it is supposed to, your body is ready, your baby is fully mature and ready to make their entrance into the world, and you naturally go into labor.

In determining if labor induction is necessary, you and your doctor or midwife will be taking several factors into consideration. Some of these include your health, the health of your baby, your baby's gestational age and size, your baby's position in the uterus, and whether your cervix is dilated or effaced.

There are several reasons your care provider could recommend an induction. The most common is if you are approaching two weeks past your due date, and labor has not started naturally. Many hospitals have a policy of induction at 10 days after the expected due date, and many birth centers require you go into labor within 42 weeks. If you reach the limit set by your care provider they may recommend an induction. Some additional reasons your doctor or midwife could recommend an induction are:

Your water has broken, but you're not having contractions. When your amniotic sac ruptures before labor begins, it is called premature rupture of membranes. It is the policy of many hospitals that when your water breaks you have 24 hours for labor to begin before they will want to induce labor. The reason for this is that you are at an increased risk for infection once your amniotic sac has ruptured.

There's not enough amniotic fluid surrounding your baby. This condition is called oligohydramnios. During pregnancy a sac filled with liquid called amniotic fluid surrounds your baby. Amniotic fluid helps protects your baby and the umbilical cord from trauma and infection. Your levels of amniotic fluid will fluctuate, depending on how hydrated you are, how much your baby swallows and urinates, and your baby's kidney function. The levels of amniotic fluid are measured using an ultrasound. If your care provider determines that your amniotic fluid levels are too low then you may be diagnosed with oligohydramnios. Please know that this happens to a very small percentage, about 4%, of pregnant women. This number does increase to about 12% in women whose pregnancies go two weeks past their due date, because the amniotic fluid usually starts decreasing at this time (March of Dimes, 2011).

Your care provider suspects you are having a large baby. There are many reasons why some babies are larger than others. This can be due to genetics or to underlying health issues like gestational diabetes. There is no way to measure a baby's size and weight accurately before birth. These measurements are usually taken with an ultrasound and they are not 100% accurate. The medical term for a big baby is macrosomia. Most guidelines consider a baby to be big if they weigh over 4,500 grams, or 9 pounds 15 ounces. The main concern with birthing a big baby is the risk of shoulder dystocia, which happens when your baby's shoulders become stuck. Shoulder dystocia is regarded as an emergency, with the potential to cause injury to your baby.

In cases of gestational diabetes, the evidence recommending induction before 41 weeks to avoid a big baby is weak. The World Health Organization does not recommend induction for gestational diabetes unless the condition is not controlled or if the placenta is not providing enough nourishment to your baby.

Intrauterine Growth Restriction (IUGR) At Term, which means your baby is small for their gestational age. Just as with a big baby, this can be due to genetics. Some babies are just small and some have restricted growth because they are not receiving enough nourishment from the placenta. Again, as with big babies, these measurements are taken with an ultrasound and it is not 100% accurate, and it relies on accurate dating of your due date. Ultrasounds during pregnancy are more accurate before 20 weeks, when the margin of error is 7-10 days; the margin for error later can be closer to 3 weeks.

Some additional reasons for an induction can be that you have a medical condition that might put you or your baby at risk, such as high blood pressure or diabetes, if there is an infection in your uterus, if your baby has stopped growing at the expected pace, or if your placenta has begun to deteriorate.

The last reason for an induction could be pure choice or convenience. Perhaps you live far from the hospital or birthing center, you have a history of really fast deliveries, or you prefer to give birth with a specific practitioner. In these cases your care provider should confirm that your baby's gestational age is at least 39 weeks, preferably 40. This is really critical because making sure your little one is full term helps reduce risks of health problems for them. Any decision to induce labor should be discussed with your doctor or midwife in detail to weigh any potential risks with the benefits.

There are multiple methods for inducing labor. Your doctor or midwife can strip or sweep the amniotic membranes. To do this your care provider inserts their gloved finger beyond your cervical opening and rotates it to separate the amniotic sac from the wall of your uterus. This doesn't actually induce labor, but it might speed the beginning of spontaneous labor, especially if your cervix has already started to dilate. This procedure can cause some intense cramping and spotting and if you leave your care provider's office and bleeding becomes heavier than a normal menstrual period, you will definitely want to contact your doctor or midwife right away.

Another method to induce is to ripen your cervix. There are a couple of ways this can be done. With a synthetic prostaglandin, which is taken orally or placed inside your vagina, or a mechanical dilator is used to physically open your cervix.

There are two basic types of prostaglandins, misoprostol (known under the brand name Cytotec) and dinoprostone (which goes by the trade names Cervidil and Prepidil). Both medications ripen the cervix, meaning they cause it to efface or thin, and cause uterine contractions. After prostaglandin use, your care provider will initially monitor your contractions and your baby's heart rate.

Misoprostol was originally approved as a medication to prevent ulcers. While it is commonly used for labor induction today, especially in the United States, it does not technically have approval from the FDA for this use (U.S. Food and Drug Administration, 2015). In the U.S. the use of Misoprostol to induce labor is off label, meaning it is not technically approved for that use, and warnings about risks associated with its use for induction of labor remain on the label. When it is used to induce it is effective at causing uterine contractions and ripening of the cervix.

The other prostaglandin used to induce labor is dinoprostone, which goes by the trade names Cervidil and Prepidil. Similar to Misoprostol it also softens the cervix and causes uterine contractions. The FDA approves dinoprostone for labor induction.

Risks associated with the use of prostaglandins include uterine hyperstimulation, which means it over stimulates your uterus to contract too much, and maternal side effects such as nausea, vomiting, diarrhea, and fever.

In comparing the two prostaglandin options, many studies show Misoprostol compared with dinoprostone appears to show less oxytocin augmentation for labor induction at term. In plain terms, less people required synthetic oxytocin during their labor after using misoprostol. The other outcomes of both drugs, like APGAR scores and C-section rates were similar. However, these findings were based on small-scale trials. Further studies assessing the effectiveness and safety of misoprostol and dinoprostone in selected groups of patients are warranted (Wang L., 2015).

There is documented concern of risks associated with misoprostol (Cytotec) that include hyperstimulating the uterus, prolonged contractions, postpartum hemorrhage, and uterine rupture among many others. Ina May Gaskin, who is perhaps the most respected figure in midwifery, wrote a strong and emotional article against the use of misoprostol (Gaskin, Cytotec and the FDA, 2013).

If you opt to induce labor with a mechanical dilator, one option is to use a small balloon-tipped catheter that is inserted beyond your cervical opening. Then saline is injected through the catheter, which expands the balloon, and causes your cervix to widen. The other option is a laminaria, which are small rods made from seaweed that are inserted into your cervix and absorb moisture and get thicker, which opens your cervix. Both of these procedures can cause some cramping.

Another method you care provider can use is to break your water. This is also known as an amniotomy or rupturing the membranes. An amniotomy is typically done only if the cervix is partially dilated and thinned and your baby's head is deep in the pelvis. Your doctor or midwife does this by making a small opening in the amniotic sac with a thin plastic hook. When this happens you may feel a warm gush of fluid when the sac opens. If your care provider ruptures your membranes they will monitor your baby's heart rate both before and after the procedure, as well as examine the amniotic fluid for traces of fecal waste, known as meconium.

When you naturally go into labor the hormone oxytocin is responsible for causing contractions. There is a synthetic version of this, most commonly known by the brand name Pitocin, which is most effective at inducing labor if your cervix has already begun to dilate and thin. This is given through an IV. Your care provider may also recommend Pitocin to augment or stimulate contractions if your labor is not progressing as quickly as they would like. With the use of Pitocin your care provider will monitor your contractions and your baby's heart rate will be continuously monitored. Synthetic oxytocin can make labor contractions really strong and lower your baby's heart rate. This is why continuous fetal monitoring is used with this method. It should also be noted that the amount of synthetic oxytocin you are administered could be adjusted so if you do go this route you can start off with a low dose, then gradually increase it if necessary.

Keep in mind that your care provider may also recommend a combination of methods to induce labor. The length of time between an induction and going into labor will depend on how you respond to the procedure. If your cervix needs to ripen, it could take a couple of days before labor starts. If your cervix has begun to soften, efface, and dilate, it could be as quick as a few hours.

The use of induction of labor has increased in the United States concurrently with the increase in cesarean delivery rates. In 1990 9.5% of births were induced and in 2008 this number rose to 23.1%. Because women who undergo induction of labor have higher rates of cesarean delivery than those who experience spontaneous labor, it has been widely assumed that induction of labor itself increases the risk of cesarean delivery. According to the American Congress of Obstetricians and Gynecologists this is not the case. Studies that compare induction of labor to its actual alternative, expectant management awaiting spontaneous labor, have found either no difference or a decreased risk of cesarean delivery among women who are induced (Caughey A.B., 2014).

If an induction is not successful your care provider may suggest a cesarean section. If you and your baby are not showing signs of distress cesarean delivery may be avoided by allowing longer duration of induction or oxytocin before deeming the induction a failure. If you do have an induction and you are not going into labor, be sure to discuss all options with your doctor or midwife and find out if you can hold off on a C-section, if that is your preference.

Although there is some disagreement as to whether induction increases your chance of a cesarean there are some other risks involved.

Inducing labor too early might result in a premature birth. This poses risks for your baby, such as respiratory issues. This is why it is so critical to be accurate with your due date. If you schedule an induction and your due date is off by a week or 2, your baby may not be full term. When babies are born prematurely they are at greater risk of respiratory problems, low blood sugar, jaundice, irregular heart rate and the inability to stabilize temperature. They are also more likely to have difficulty with establishing breastfeeding.

Medications used to induce labor — synthetic oxytocin or a prostaglandin — might provoke too many contractions, which can diminish your baby's oxygen supply and lower your baby's heart rate.

Your baby and your uterus are protected from infection by the amniotic sac. Once this breaks, germs like bacteria can get in more easily and cause an infection, so rupturing your membranes increases your risk for infection.

Labor induction increases the risk of the umbilical cord prolapse, which happens when the umbilical cord slips into the vagina before your baby, which can compress the cord and decrease your baby's supply of oxygen, which can be a serious complication.

Uterine rupture is a rare but serious complication in which the uterus tears open along the scar line from a prior C-section or major uterine surgery, which causes heavy bleeding. In these cases an emergency C-section is done to prevent life-threatening complications.

Labor induction increases the risk of uterine atony, which occurs when your uterine muscles don't properly contract after you give birth, and this can cause hemorrhage after delivery.

For more information on induction you can listen to episode 20 of the Pregnancy Podcast at PregnancyPodcast.com/episode20.

There are some ways you can try to induce labor naturally. Before you attempt any method you want to make sure your care provider is on board and that you are confident your due date is correct. Do not attempt to naturally induce labor until your due date or longer. Any form of induction is an induction, even if it is something you are doing at home, and you wouldn't want to jump start labor unless your body is ready and your baby is full term. Keep in mind, the only surefire way to go into labor naturally is to wait it out and let your baby and your body tell you when it is time.

If you would like to find out more about inducing labor naturally you can listen to Episode 21 of the Pregnancy Podcast at PregnancyPodcast.com/episode21.

Electronic Fetal Monitoring

During your labor your doctor or midwife will be checking the heartbeat of your baby. This is monitored because your little one's heart rate is thought of as the best way to check their well being during labor. Your baby's normal heart rate can be anywhere between about 110 to 160 beats per minute, and their heart rate is constantly changing. This constant changing is referred to as the variability or beat-to-beat variation. A healthy beat-to-beat variation is generally at least five beats per minute. Your baby's heartbeat will speed up, which is known as fetal heart accelerations, when they move in the womb, when your doctor or midwife is feeling your belly and putting pressure on it to determine where your baby is, or if their head is touched during a vaginal exam. You can see that some variations are common and are no big deal. Detecting an abnormal fetal heart rate does not always mean there is a problem.

Labor and birth is going to be the most stressful event of your baby's life, and the reason for this is that each time you have a contraction, the blood flow to the placenta is temporarily diminished and this reduces your baby's oxygen supply. This might sound a little scary, but this is totally normal. This is how we are designed to work, and our babies are designed to cope with this. The decrease in oxygen supply to the placenta is short and the oxygen supply will increase as soon as your contraction is over. When you have a contraction and the supply of oxygen to the placenta is reduced your baby's heart rate slows down, and then returns to their normal heart rate after the contraction is over.

There are some instances in which your baby's oxygen supply can be reduced too much which can compromise their health and well-being, this situation is referred to as fetal distress and is detected by significant changes in their heart rate. The goal of using electronic fetal monitoring is to identify babies who are short on oxygen and identify what the underlying cause is to correct it. Monitoring heart rate can also alert your doctor or midwife in the event an emergency arises in which your baby needs to be born immediately either via cesarean section or through an assisted birth.

The method of monitoring your baby's heart rate depends on your doctor or midwife, the policy of the venue where you are giving birth, your risk of complications, and how your labor is going. There are two methods that can be used to monitor your baby's heart rate; monitoring is done either through auscultation or electronic fetal monitoring.

Auscultation is a method of periodically listening to your baby's heartbeat. This is usually done with a Doppler transducer, but your care provider may also use a fetal stethoscope, or a Pinard, which is a trumpet shaped device that amplifies sound. In most cases a Doppler is used and this device is shaped like a microphone and when it is held up to your belly you can hear the heartbeat amplified through a speaker. Chances are you have seen this at one of your prenatal appointments. As long as everything is going fine during your labor your care provider will be checking this from time to time. In general with intermittent monitoring they will be checking about every 15 minutes during the first stage of labor, when you are dilating. During the second stage of labor, or the pushing stage, they will be checking more frequently, generally about every five minutes. This could be more frequent; ultimately it is up to your care provider to decide how often they want to check your baby's heart rate.

Electronic fetal monitoring uses instruments to continuously record the heartbeat of your baby and the contractions of the uterus during labor. The machine used is a cardiotocograph, or CTG, and more commonly known as an electronic fetal monitor. This provides an ongoing record so your care provider can go back and look at the results of how your contractions and your baby's heartbeat have changed over time. This record can either be a print out or show up and be recorded on a screen.

Electronic Fetal Monitoring can be external, internal, or both. With external monitoring a pair of belts is wrapped around your abdomen. One of the belts is using a Doppler to detect your baby's heart rate, and the other belt measures the length of contractions and the time between contractions. This is by far the most common method of monitoring. It is not considered invasive because the belts are just strapped around your belly but you will be connected via wires to the CTG machine so you may not be able to move or walk around too much. There are some instances in which external monitoring is not working well or if your doctor or midwife has some concern and wants a more accurate reading and may recommend internal monitoring.

With internal monitoring a wire, called an electrode, is placed on the part of your baby closest to your cervix, usually their scalp, and this records the heart rate. There is a tiny screw that is used to hold it in place. Your contractions may also be monitored intermittently by using an intrauterine pressure catheter. Which is a tube that is inserted into your uterus, through your vagina. Internal monitoring is only used after your water has broken, and you are dilated at least 1-3 centimeters. One reason for internal monitoring could be that you are having twins, in which they want to make sure they can differentiate the heartbeat of each baby, usually referred to as baby A and baby B. Another reason for internal monitoring is if mom is significantly overweight in which case it can be tough to detect a heartbeat with an external monitor. Internal monitoring is not a routine procedure and your care provider will only be using this if there is cause to do so. With internal monitoring there is a slight risk of infection and the possibility that the electrode can cause bruising on your baby. There may also be some discomfort when the electrode is put in your uterus. There are some instances in which internal monitoring is not recommended and this would be if you are HIV positive or if you have an active herpes infection. With internal monitoring you will be required to stay in bed and will not be able to move around very much.

If you are having a home birth or a birth center birth, you will be monitored intermittently via auscultation, and not with a CTG machine. If you are having your baby at a hospital you may have some options about how you are monitored and whether it is intermittent or continuous. Some reasons your care provider may prefer continuous monitoring are if you get an epidural, have Pitocin, which is synthetic oxytocin to induce or augment your labor, or if you are high-risk or incur any complications. A few examples of things that could make a pregnancy high-risk include diabetes or high blood pressure, or if your baby is not developing or growing as well as they should be.

Electronic fetal monitoring is often continuous but it doesn't necessarily have to be as long as you and baby are doing well. Ultimately this is something you will need to discuss with your care provider. If you are having a hospital birth you will probably be hooked up to a monitor for about 20-30 minutes once you arrive at the hospital in labor. If everything is going well, you may be able to have the belts removed and hook it up intermittently. There is some research that there is no evidence of benefit for the use of an electronic fetal monitor upon admission to a hospital when in labor and admission CTG increases the cesarean section rate by approximately 20%. The findings of this review support recommendations that the admission CTG not be used for women who are low-risk on admission in labor and goes on to recommend that women should be informed that admission CTG is likely associated with an increase in the incidence of cesarean section without evidence of benefit (Devane D., 2012).

One big issue with electronic fetal monitoring and continuous monitoring is that it impacts your ability to move around because you are tethered to a machine with wires. One other option you may have is telemetry monitoring. A telemetry monitor uses a transmitter on your thigh to transmit your baby's heartbeat via radio waves. It is usually transmitted to a nurse's station so you can be walking around and have much more mobility while you are in labor and still have constant monitoring. Not all hospitals will have a telemetry monitor available but if it is something you are interested in you can ask your care provider if this is an option. This would allow you much more mobility than a standard CTG machine.

If you are being monitored electronically there is a volume dial on an electronic monitoring machine. If you find it distracting you can always turn the volume down, or even turn the monitor away so you are not looking at it. You want your partner paying attention to you not the machine and if it is a distraction to them you can turn it down or turn it away. If you are listening to the heart rate and it suddenly stops, do not panic. The transducer probably shifted out of place and a nurse or your care provider should be able to adjust it. If you are paying attention to the machine don't stress out if there are changes in your baby's heart rate. Some changes are completely normal so don't focus 100% of your energy on trying to be a pro at reading the results of the monitor.

A review of 13 trials and over 37,000 women compared intermittent monitoring with continuous monitoring and found overall, there was no difference in the number of babies who died during or shortly after labor. Neonatal seizures in babies are very rare, but they occurred significantly less often when continuous monitoring was used. There was no difference in the incidence of cerebral palsy. The research showed that continuous monitoring was associated with a significant increase in cesarean section and instrumental vaginal births (Alfirevic Z., 2013).

Electronic fetal monitoring is almost always used in situations where your baby is considered high-risk. This makes sense on the surface but there is no hard evidence that continuous electronic fetal monitoring has improved outcomes for babies in high-risk pregnancies (Grivell R.M., 2015).

For more information on electronic fetal monitoring you can listen to episode 35 of the Pregnancy Podcast at PregnancyPodcast.com/episode35.

IV Fluids

Most hospitals require a saline lock, sometimes called a hep-lock. This is an IV catheter that is put in on the top of your hand. The needle is taped in place with a small tube that is capped off. With a hep-lock in you are not hooked up to an IV pole. In the event you needed something intravenously your care provider can simply connect an IV tube to the hep-lock. There are several reasons why an IV might be used in labor and birth. The most common reason your care provider will put you on an IV is to keep you hydrated. Staying hydrated during labor sounds great on the surface but this can also cause edema, which is swelling due to excess fluids in your body.

IV fluids can also cause your baby to maintain higher fluid levels at birth, leading to more excess fluid loss after birth, which your care provider may interpret as weight loss due to not eating enough. Often this results in a fear that your baby is not getting enough nutrition from breastfeeding and formula may be started when it is not necessary. An observational study published in the International Breastfeeding Journal found that timing and amounts of maternal IV fluids are correlated to newborn weight loss (Noel-Weiss J., 2011). The authors of this study recommend using the 24-hour weight, rather than the weight at birth, as the baseline weight when following infant weight over time. This recommendation has not gained traction in the medical community. This may be something to keep in mind if you receive IV fluids during labor.

In the past, hospitals discouraged drinking and eating during labor. This practice is improving with most care providers supporting consumption of food and drinking water at least during the first stage of labor. Midwives at birth centers and attending home births often encourage you to eat and drink. Labor is a marathon and you need to stay hydrated. If you want to avoid IV fluids make sure you are hydrated and drink water or eat lots of ice chips. If you do receive an IV most IV poles have wheels so you can walk around and can still maintain some mobility.

Antibiotics (Group B Strep)

Group B streptococcus (GBS) is a type of bacterial infection. This bacterium naturally lives in the gastrointestinal tract and is present in the vagina and/or rectum of about 25% of all healthy women. This bacterium can come and go, and once you have it that does not mean you will always have it. Most women who are colonized with group B strep do not experience any symptoms, and normally this is not a big deal. It can become an issue when you are pregnant and there is a possibility of passing group B strep to your baby. GBS can cause bladder and uterine infections for you and in serious cases; GBS can cause meningitis, sepsis, pneumonia, or stillbirth.

Group B strep can be a serious complication for a newborn baby. There are two types of infections that could affect your baby, early or late-onset GBS. Early-onset GBS is the most common and symptoms usually show up within a few hours after birth and can include sepsis, pneumonia, and meningitis, which are the most common complications. GBS can also cause breathing problems, heart and blood pressure instability, and gastrointestinal and kidney problems. Late-onset GBS usually show up within a week up to three months after birth and the most common symptom is meningitis. Late-onset GBS could have resulted from GBS being passed from mom to baby, or your baby could possibly contract it from coming into contact with someone who was colonized. This section is focused on early-onset.

If you do have GBS that does not mean that your baby will have it also. GBS is passed from mom to baby during birth, and there are some things that can be done to prevent your baby from being colonized. In the United States about 1 in every 2,000 babies is affected by GBS. Of mothers who carry GBS, without treatment, approximately 1 out of every 200 babies will be affected. With treatment this drops to 1 in 4,000.

Testing for GBS during pregnancy has become routine because it can be a dangerous complication. The test for GBS is done between week 35 and 37. This isn't done earlier because it is possible that you could test negative early on, but that it would be present later in your pregnancy and at birth. Your care provider wants to know if you are colonized during labor, which is when it could potentially be passed to your baby. This is a non-invasive test and your care provider will take a swab of your vagina and rectum, then the sample is sent to a lab where a culture is analyzed for the presence of GBS. Results should be available within 24 to 48 hours.

If the results of your group B strep test are negative then there is nothing to worry about, if the result is positive, you and your care provider will be taking some precautions. You will be considered to be at a higher risk of passing it to your baby if you go into labor or your water breaks before week 37, if your water breaks more than 18 hours before your baby is born, if you have a fever during labor, if you have a urinary tract infection as a result of GBS, or if you had a previous baby with GBS.

In the U.S. it is common practice to treat a mother with antibiotics if they are colonized with group B strep, even if she is considered low-risk. Without antibiotics there is a 50% chance your baby would become colonized, and with antibiotics, that drops significantly. Antibiotics are given to you in the beginning of your labor through an IV, then every four hours during active labor until your baby is born. The reason you don't get antibiotics before you are in labor is that since GBS lives in your gastrointestinal tract, it could potentially come back after antibiotics, but before you give birth. The antibiotic most commonly used is penicillin, if you have an allergy to penicillin there are a few other antibiotics that may be given and you can talk to your care provider about alternatives.

GBS is normally not passed to your baby if you are having a cesarean section. If your water breaks, the chances of an infection are higher and antibiotics may be recommended, even if you are planning a cesarean section.

Getting antibiotics does not necessarily mean that you will be continuously hooked up to an IV. Once your labor starts you will have an IV put in and it takes about 15-30 minutes. The antibiotics are only given every 4 hours until birth, and for many women this is only once or twice. In between getting intravenous antibiotics you can have a help-lock in, which means the needle stays in your hand, but it is capped off and disconnected from the IV tubes. This allows you to be able to move around without being hooked up to tubes and an IV pole.

Antibiotics given to you during labor will cross the placenta and enter your baby. The big question is what impact is this going to have on your baby? Group B strep is pretty serious and your number one priority is making sure your baby doesn't get a group B strep infection. At birth, your baby's gastrointestinal tract is sterile, and bacteria originating from both you and their environment rapidly colonize. If you have any concerns about how antibiotics could affect the gut microbiome of your little one, there is a lot you can do to help make sure they do have a healthy gut. One of the best things you can do for this is to breastfeed. If you have concerns, definitely discuss them with your care provider. If you and your care provider decide the best course of action is for you to have antibiotics to protect your baby from a serious infection, that will likely outweigh concerns of your baby's gut bacteria in the short term.

There is some interesting research that taking a probiotic may decrease your risk for group B strep. Our bodies are a really complex system with a lot of different bacteria. 25% of pregnant women are colonized with group b streptococcus. This is just one of a ton of different bacterium living in our bodies. A study done with the effects of lactobacilli, which is another bacteria, found that high numbers of lactobacilli in women may contribute to a low vaginal pH and seems to have a negative influence on group B streptococci. This particular study used panty liners to introduce lactobacilli to the participants (Rönnqvist P.D., 2006). You might be grossed out by the thought of using a panty liner colonized with bacteria, but there is a much easier way to introduce lactobacilli to your body.

A very small study found that a prenatal probiotic has the potential to reduce GBS colonization (Hanson L., 2014). This study was significant because it justified a controlled clinical trial. At the time of this writing Stanford University is in the middle of a clinical trial with the purpose of determining if oral probiotic supplementation during the second half of pregnancy decreases maternal GBS colonization. The importance of this study is that it may offer a safer alternative to antibiotic treatment of GBS colonized pregnant women. Final results of the study are not expected until 2018 (Stanford University, 2014).

You are already taking a prenatal vitamin; it wouldn't be a big deal to add a probiotic. It doesn't need to be a fancy or expensive probiotic but you do want to look for one that has lactobacillus, and most will. In the small study mentioned above no women reported any negative effects from taking a daily probiotic, and half reported improved gastrointestinal symptoms (Rönnqvist P.D., 2006). Yes of course it is possible that you still end up with GBS, but it is also possible that you could prevent it.

For more information on group B strep you can listen to episode 43 of the Pregnancy podcast at PregnancyPodcast.com/episode43.

Epidural

The term epidural is commonly used to encompass any type of anesthetic medication used for labor and birth. There are actually three separate procedures that can be done that are often lumped under the umbrella term, "epidural". The three procedures are epidurals, spinals, and the combined spinal epidural.

An epidural blocks the nerve impulses from the lower spinal segments. The end result is decreased sensation in the lower half of the body, with continuous delivery of medication. A tiny catheter is in inserted into a space between your vertebrae. Once it is in place, medication is delivered through the thin tube. It will take around 15 minutes to work and if more medication is needed or wanted, more can be delivered.

A spinal is a one-time injection directly into your spinal fluid. This is also sometimes called a spinal block, and there is no continuous medication being delivered. This gets to work pretty quickly, usually within about 5 minutes, but it will only last an hour or two.

A spinal is frequently used in conjunction with an epidural to make a combined spinal epidural. This takes effect within about five minutes, like a spinal and then works to deliver continuous medication like an epidural.

For the purposes of this section we are talking about an epidural as in the catheter in your back delivering continuous medication whether that is solely an epidural or the combination of a spinal and epidural. If you want to get into more detail as to your options between just an epidural and a combined spinal epidural you will need to talk to your care provider. While they do differ, both are delivering continuous medication. With an epidural an initial dose of narcotic, anesthetic, or a combination of the two is injected, then the anesthesiologist will pull the needle back into the epidural space, thread a catheter through the needle, then withdraw the needle and leave the catheter in place. Epidurals are common and in the United States over 60% of moms who have a vaginal birth receive an epidural (Osterman M.J.K., 2011).

The medications used for an epidural can be a combination of more than one drug. What medications are used, in what amounts, and for how long will all depend on your individual needs, your care provider, and the hospital. Different techniques, medications and doses all have different results and risks, so it is really important to talk to your care provider about what their policy and practices are. Knowing what your medication options are lets you make the best choice for you and your baby. Generally, the medication you will receive is a combination of a local anesthetic used to decrease feeling in a specific area, like bupivacaine, chloroprocaine, or lidocaine, and an opioid like fentanyl or morphine, which decreases the required dose of the anesthetic and prolongs the effect, while stabilizing your blood pressure. The end result is relief from feeling contractions with minimal effects. Depending on the hospital and where you live, additional drugs could be added to an epidural. In the U.K. diamorphine is also added to an epidural for a cesarean section. If you are not familiar with diamorphine, it is medical grade heroin. When you are talking about medications via an epidural you are dealing with some powerful and very effective drugs.

An epidural will almost always come along with IV fluids and continuous electronic fetal monitoring. If you know that you want an epidural but would like to minimize IV fluids or electronic fetal monitoring, you may have limited options. Talk to your care provider and find out what their policy and recommendation is.

A walking epidural is really just a lower dose of medication from a combined spinal epidural that allows you to maintain more feeling. You may not necessarily be able to actually walk around with this. Also you will likely be hooked up with the epidural in your back, an IV delivering fluids through a tube in the top of your hand, and an electronic fetal monitor strapped to your belly so you will have limited mobility, even if you do feel enough sensation to stand up. A lower dose of medication and more sensation means it may be easier to feel when you are having a contraction or when you need to push during the second stage of labor.

An option you may have access to is patient-controlled epidural analgesia. Patient controlled means a pump is connected to the epidural that has a button you can push if you would like more medication. This gives you more control over the amount of medication you are receiving. You don't need to worry about overdosing because the pump is going to be preprogrammed with limits on how much medication can be delivered.

Depending on how numb you are with an epidural you may have difficulty telling when you are having a contraction and this can make pushing difficult to control. A review of 38 different studies involving nearly 1,000 women shows that an epidural tends to make the second "pushing" stage of labor longer (Anim-Somuah M., 2011). If you are having a tough time pushing during the second stage of labor it is possible that your little one needs some assistance and a vacuum or forceps will be used. Women who get an epidural are at an increased risk for an instrumental or assisted delivery, and this almost always comes with an episiotomy.

In the past, many doctors wanted you to be in active labor before starting an epidural. The concern was that an epidural might slow down your contractions. Today, many care providers will allow you to start an epidural whenever you ask for it. Talk to your care provider about when you can get an epidural this so you know what their policy is. If you know the second you get to the hospital you're going to want an epidural, you can ask the anesthesiologist to put the catheter in place once you are settled into the delivery room, and you can always wait to start the medication when your labor becomes more active. You also have the option to hold off, which could be beneficial if being more mobile is helpful for you. Your mobility will be more limited with IVs, an epidural, and fetal monitoring. You can get an epidural up until your baby's head is crowning. It is very unlikely, especially if this is your first baby, that you will get to that point in a super short period of time.

Aside from the obvious of not feeling the discomfort of contractions there can be some benefits to an epidural. First, having an epidural can allow you to rest. This could be a big benefit if you have had a particularly long labor. Another benefit is that an epidural does not knock you out, so you will still be alert and be an active participant in your birth. As your needs change during labor, the type, amounts, and strength of the medications can be adjusted. To minimize feeling contractions during labor an epidural is the most widely used, and the most effective, medication and delivery system available today.

As with any medication there are possible side effects that you might experience. A few of these are shivering, ringing in your ears, backache, or soreness where the needle is inserted. The narcotics delivered through an epidural can cause itchiness, particularly in your face. The medications used could also make you nauseous, although keep in mind you could also be nauseous from labor without an epidural. An epidural can make it difficult to tell when you need to urinate, and you could end up with a catheter to empty your bladder. About 14 out of every 100 women who get an epidural end up with a catheter. An epidural raises your risk of running a fever in labor, which affects about 23 out of 100 women (Institute for Quality and Efficiency in Health Care, 2012). Unfortunately we do not know exactly why this happens. Having a fever does not increase your risk or your baby's risk of an infection, but since a fever is a sign of an infection, it is possible you or your baby could end up with antibiotics unnecessarily. An epidural may cause your blood pressure to suddenly drop; this happens in about 14 every 100 women (Institute for Quality and Efficiency in Health Care, 2012). The issue with your blood pressure dropping is that it also affects blood flow to your baby. A drop in blood pressure is often treated with IV fluids, medications, and oxygen. One side effect that affects about 1 in 100 women who receive an epidural is a severe headache, which is caused by leakage of spinal fluid

(Institute for Quality and Efficiency in Health Care, 2012). This can be treated with a procedure called a "blood patch", in which a small amount of your blood is injected into the epidural space. You can reduce the risk of headache by lying as still as possible during the procedure while the needle is being placed. In rare instances an epidural could affect your breathing and very rarely could cause permanent nerve damage or result in an infection. This is an overview of the side effects and this list is not specific to particular medications so you definitely want to discuss any possible side effects of the specific medications you will be given with your care provider.

There are no perfect studies with controlled test groups and it is tough to assess exactly what the impact of an epidural on your baby is. Any medication that you use during labor enters your baby's bloodstream through the umbilical cord. Many of the effects on your baby are a direct result of the possible side effects the epidural can have on you, like running a fever or having a drop in your blood pressure. The research available indicates epidurals have no known long-term disadvantages, but more studies and research are really needed.

The research on epidurals and their impact on breastfeeding is a little tough to dissect. The studies are about split in half between those that showed a negative association between epidurals and breastfeeding and about half of the studies showing no effect (French C.A., 2016). It is really difficult to pinpoint a correlation between one intervention, like an epidural, with an outcome, like breastfeeding, because there are so many other variables. If you are planning on an epidural and you are concerned about your baby breastfeeding take advantage of being in a hospital and ask to see a lactation consultant to really make sure you get off on the right foot with breastfeeding.

Much of the data on epidurals shows an increase for fetal malposition, meaning the baby is in a "face-up" position at delivery; this usually makes for a longer labor, higher doses of Pitocin, and a significantly higher rate of C-sections. Epidurals are also associated with a longer second stage of labor, and fetal distress (Osterman M.J.K., 2011).

If you are planning on getting an epidural or have any questions about it talk to your care provider. Some questions you can ask them are:
What combination and what dosage of drugs will be used?
What are the potential side effects of these drugs?
What are your policies for procedures like an assisted delivery if an epidural creates a need for it?
How can the medications affect my baby?
Will I be able to get up and walk around or how could my mobility could be impacted?

Are there any restrictions of what liquids and solids I can eat or drink during labor?

For more information on epidurals you can listen to episode 38 of the Pregnancy Podcast at PregnancyPodcast.com/episode38.

Episiotomy

It is fairly common for first time mothers to have some tearing during a vaginal delivery. There is also the possibility that you could have an episiotomy. The tear or incision is to your perineum, which is the spot between your vaginal opening and your anus. Although all of this can sound scary, the benefits of a vaginal delivery far outweigh the downside of a tear or an episiotomy.

To state the obvious, when your baby is born your vagina has to stretch so they can come out. Generally they are head first, and their head is the biggest part, once their head is out the rest of their body comes pretty easily. This happens in the second stage of labor, which is the pushing stage. Keep in mind, your body and these parts are made to stretch. Humans have been giving birth for a really long time, the equipment we have works, and it was made to do this. Unfortunately, sometimes when your skin is stretching during birth it can tear. This tends to be common with first time moms, and is less of an issue in subsequent births. There are some cases where your care provider may recommend an episiotomy. An episiotomy is a surgical cut a doctor or midwife makes to the opening of the vagina during the last stages of childbirth, when your baby is coming out.

The good news is that there are some things you can do leading up to, and during, your labor and delivery to help prevent tearing. If you prevent tearing, you will also prevent an episiotomy.

Perineal massage is one thing you can do, and you can start doing this at home after week 34 of your pregnancy. To get started, you want to wash your hands and you will be using a mild lubricant, like K-Y jelly, almond oil, or coconut oil, to name a few options. You put the lubricant on your thumbs and place your thumbs just inside your vagina and you are going to press downward toward your rectum. When you do this you hold for one to two minutes, then, you slowly massage the lower half of your vagina. You are going to repeat the massage for about 10 minutes, every day until delivery.

Applying a warm compress or warm oil to your perineum helps increase blood flow to the area, and softens the tissue and the muscles there. This can help prevent tearing. If you are considering a water birth, the warm water should help soften the tissue to prevent a tear. Applying oil might be a little difficult for you to do yourself during labor so you want to enlist the help of your partner, your doula, a nurse, your midwife, or your doctor.

Using a lubricant, like a warmed mineral oil, can help to decrease friction and help your baby slide out a little bit easier. Again, this will probably be tough for you to do yourself so enlist the help of your doula, a nurse, your care provider, or even your partner.

Slow pushing is another excellent way to allow your skin time to stretch during labor. Your initial thought is probably that you want to push your baby out as quickly as possible but there are benefits to slowing down this process. To slow down pushing try exhale pushing. To do this you slowly breathe in and slowly exhale; it may also help to make a low or deep sound as you push. This will make the pushing stage a bit slower than taking a deep breath, holding it and then pushing. When your baby starts to crown, you can switch to using short, almost grunting, pushes. It can be hard to keep these techniques in mind when you are in the midst of labor. Talk about this with your partner, your doula, and any staff who will present to remind you to do this and they can help guide you through pushing.

Vaginal tears are classified by four degrees with first-degree being the most minor and fourth-degree being the most severe. First-degree tears only involve the skin around the vaginal opening or perineal skin. These usually are not very painful although you could experience some burning or stinging with urination. A first-degree tear may or may not require stitches and usually heals within a few weeks. Second-degree tears involve the perineal muscles, which are the muscles between the vagina and the anus that support your uterus, bladder, and rectum. A second-degree tear usually requires stitches and heals within a few weeks. Both first and second-degree tears are typically stitched in the delivery room with a local anesthetic. Third and fourth-degree tears involve the perineal muscles and the muscles that surround the anus, and in the case of a fourth-degree tear involve the tissue lining the rectum. These tears can require repair in an operating room, and can take months to heal. Some complications can be fecal incontinence and painful intercourse. Third and fourth-degree tears are much less common than the milder first and second-degree. Often a care provider will recommend an episiotomy if they believe it could prevent a third or fourth-degree tear.

Episiotomy has become one of the most commonly performed surgical procedures in the world, but that doesn't necessarily mean that its wide use is warranted. The Journal of the American Medical Association suggests that between 30% and 35% of vaginal births in the U.S. involve an episiotomy (Hartmann K., 2005). In other parts of the globe, rates range from 3.7% in Denmark to 75.0% in Cyprus (Blondel B. & Committee, 2016). Among midwives, who generally perform fewer interventions than a traditional physician, episiotomy rates in the U.S. are at or below 3%.

In the past, routine episiotomies were recommended. Research has shown us that routine episiotomies are not a good thing, and a better policy is restricting their use. The Journal of the American Medical Association found evidence does not support maternal benefits that were traditionally ascribed to routine episiotomy. In fact, outcomes with episiotomy can be considered worse since some proportion of women who would have had lesser injury instead had a surgical incision. Those who have an episiotomy may be more likely to have pain with intercourse in the months after pregnancy and are slower to resume having intercourse. Clinicians have been the primary agents to exercise choice to conduct or not conduct an episiotomy, rather than patients. Rates of episiotomy of less than 15% of spontaneous vaginal births should be immediately within reach. The AMA suggests episiotomies should be at 15%, but in the U.S. the rate is closer to 30% (Hartmann K., 2005).

While routine episiotomies are generally not practiced today, the procedure is warranted in some cases. Your care provider might recommend an episiotomy if extensive vaginal tearing appears likely, if your baby is in an abnormal position, if your baby is very large (as in cases of fetal macrosomia), or if an issue arises where your baby needs to be delivered quickly.

If you need an episiotomy and you haven't had any type of anesthesia or if the anesthesia has worn off, don't worry you won't feel anything. You will receive an injection of a local anesthetic to numb the tissue. You won't feel your care provider making the incision or repairing it after delivery.

There are two types of episiotomy incisions. The first is a midline or median incision, which is done vertically. This is the easiest to repair, but it has a higher risk of extending into the anal area. The second is a mediolateral incision, which is done at an angle. This offers the best protection from an extended tear going to the anal area, but is often more painful and might be more difficult to repair. Research shows that a midline incision results in deeper perineal tears, otherwise there was no statistical significant difference in the two (Sooklim R., 2007). The type of incision used is usually at the discretion of your doctor or midwife so this may be something you want to bring up ahead of time if you prefer one to the other. After an episiotomy, your care provider will repair the incision with stitches that will dissolve, and again you shouldn't feel a thing. If you do have any discomfort, be sure to ask for another local anesthetic, there is no reason for you to be in any pain during this procedure.

If your care provider uses forceps during your delivery you may benefit from an episiotomy. A study showed that in a forceps delivery, performance of an episiotomy decreases the risk of perineal tears of all degrees. When they analyzed the type of episiotomy, mediolateral incisions seemed to be more protective against perineal trauma in women undergoing forceps delivery (Bodner-Adler B., 2003).

For more information on episiotomy you can listen to episode 22 of the Pregnancy podcast at PregnancyPodcast.com/episode22.

Assisted Delivery

An assisted delivery, sometimes called an instrumental delivery, is when your doctor will help in the birthing process by using instruments such as a ventouse suction cup or forceps to help you deliver your baby. Often an assisted delivery is accompanied by an episiotomy to allow for more room for the instruments and a quicker delivery.

The word "ventouse" comes from the French word for "suction cup". A ventouse suction cup can also be referred to as vacuum-assisted vaginal delivery, or a vacuum extraction. This method uses a metal or plastic suction cup, which is placed onto the head of your baby, and the suction draws the skin from the scalp into the cup. When your baby's head is delivered, which is usually the most challenging part of delivery, the device is detached.

An alternative to a ventouse suction cup is forceps, which are a surgical instrument that resembles a pair of tongs that fit to surround your baby's head.

Any method of assisted delivery does come with risks to you or your baby. A review of 32 studies, involving over 6,500 women, compared a ventouse to forceps. The review found that forceps were more effective to achieve a vaginal birth, however, with forceps there was a trend to more cesarean sections, and significantly more third- or fourth-degree tears, this included with and without an episiotomy. There was also a higher rate of vaginal trauma, use of general anesthesia, and flatus incontinence, which is uncontrollable gas, or other continence issues. Lastly a facial injury to the baby was more likely with forceps. Among different types of ventouse, the metal cup was more likely to result in a successful vaginal birth than the soft cup, with more cases of scalp injury and cephalhematoma, which is the swelling of an infant's scalp as a result of hemorrhaging or a collection of blood. Overall forceps or the metal cup appear to be most effective at achieving a vaginal birth, but with increased risk of maternal trauma with forceps and neonatal trauma with the metal cup (O'Mahony F., 2010).

C-Sections

A cesarean section, also known as a C-section, is a surgical procedure used to deliver a baby through incisions in the mother's abdomen and uterus. A C-section could be planned ahead of time if you have a complication that would make a vaginal delivery difficult or you have had a previous C-section and aren't considering vaginal birth after cesarean (VBAC). Often a cesarean is not planned and the circumstances of your birth change when you are in labor, which lead to a C-section.

Since 1985, the international healthcare community has considered the ideal rate for cesarean sections to be between 10-15%. The World Health Organization's official stance on C-sections is that cesarean sections are effective in saving maternal and infant lives, but only when they are required for medically indicated reasons. The World Health Organization states that cesarean section rates higher than 10% are not associated with reductions in maternal and newborn mortality rates. Cesarean sections should ideally only be undertaken when medically necessary. The effects of cesarean section rates on other outcomes, such as maternal and perinatal morbidity, pediatric outcomes, and psychological or social well being are still unclear. They conclude that more research is needed to understand the health effects of cesarean section on immediate and future outcomes (Department of Reproductive Health and Research World Health Organization, 2015). There is some additional research from the Journal of the American Medical Association showing the optimal cesarean delivery rate should be closer to 19% (Molina G., 2015). Even with an optimal rate of 19%, actual C-section rates are much higher than that.

The overall cesarean delivery rate in the United States increased 60% from 1996 through 2009, from 20.7% to 32.9%. Since 2009, the cesarean rate has declined slightly, to 32.7% in 2013. Even with the decline in the C-section rate, nearly one-third of babies are delivered by this method. Of course the rate of C-sections is much higher in high-risk pregnancies but the rate of C-sections for low-risk pregnancies is still just over 1 in 4 births. Low-risk cesarean delivery is defined as a cesarean delivery for a baby at 37 weeks or more, singleton, meaning not twins or multiples, the baby is vertex, meaning they are head first, and it is the mom's first pregnancy. The rate of C-sections to low-risk women has declined in recent years, it was 32.5% in 1990, and as of 2013 was 26.5% (Osterman, 2014).

If you have a non-emergency planned C-section to take place before 39 weeks your doctor may want to test your baby's lung maturity. The last few weeks are really critical to lung development. This test is done with an amniocentesis, which uses a needle to take a sample of amniotic fluid from the uterus. There can be risks associated with an amniocentesis as it is considered an invasive test. Be sure to discuss the possible risks with your care provider.

For more information on an amniocentesis you can listen to episode 16 of the Pregnancy Podcast at PregnancyPodcast.com/episode16.

A cesarean section is going to be accompanied by a catheter and IV fluids. You can also expect to receive antibiotics through your IV. Antibiotics will help prevent infection after the operation. A review of 95 studies involving over 15,000 women found that routine use of antibiotics during cesarean section reduced the risk of infections in mothers as well as the risk of serious complications of infections by 60% to 70%. This was whether the antibiotics were given before or after clamping of the umbilical cord. The review notes that none of the studies looked properly at possible adverse effects on the baby. Although there are benefits for the mother, there is some uncertainty about whether there are any important effects on the baby (Smaill F.M., 2014). If antibiotics are given before the cord is clamped they would also go to your baby. If you have any concern about how antibiotics could affect your baby talk to your care provider and to ask them about it and find out if it is their practice to administer antibiotics before or after clamping the umbilical cord.

The majority of C-sections are done with an epidural or a spinal block that numbs just the lower part of your body. With a spinal or epidural, or a combination of the two, you remain awake and alert during the procedure. These types of medications are extremely effective and you will not feel any pain during the procedure, but you may still feel some pressure or a tugging sensation during the surgery. In an emergency scenario, you could be put under general anesthesia, which knocks you out. In this case you would not be able to see, feel or hear anything during the birth. General anesthesia is not routine and should only be used if absolutely necessary.

If you would like your partner to be present during the surgery they should be able to be there, assuming there isn't an emergency and you are not under general anesthesia. They will get to put on a lovely operating room outfit and will be seated by your head so they are not watching the actual procedure, but will be right there by your side to meet your baby.

The process of a cesarean section can vary depending on your individual circumstances but overall the procedure is going to take about 45 minutes to an hour. In this time, your baby is usually delivered in the first 5-15 minutes, and the remainder of the time is used for closing the incision. This procedure will be done in an operating room by an OB-GYN.

The procedure is going to start with cleaning your abdomen and your doctor making an incision through your abdominal wall. The incision is most commonly done horizontally near the pubic hairline, and this is known as a bikini incision. If the circumstances require that your baby needs to be delivered very quickly, a vertical incision can be used and this is from just below your navel to just above the pubic bone. The incisions are going to be made layer by layer, these will go through your fatty tissue and connective tissue and separate the abdominal muscle to access your abdominal cavity. Next, an incision is made into the uterus. This incision could be horizontal or vertical, and it does not have to be the same type of incision made in your abdomen. The most commonly used uterine incision is a low transverse incision, similar to the bikini incision. This has fewer risks and complications than the other types of incisions and it may allow you to attempt a VBAC, or a vaginal birth after cesarean, in your next pregnancy with little risk of uterine rupture. Another option for the type of incision is a classical incision, which is made vertically. A classical incision is usually reserved for complicated situations such as placenta previa, extreme emergencies, or for babies with abnormalities.

Your doctor will put up a screen above your waist so you are not watching the surgery take place. If you want to see the actual moment your baby comes out you can request that your doctor or a nurse lowers the screen slightly so you can see your baby. They probably will not remove the screen entirely, but they should be able to lower it a bit.

Once all of the incisions are made, your baby is going to be ready to make their big entrance into the world. Your doctor will suction out the amniotic fluid and then deliver your baby. Your baby's head will be delivered first and your doctor will clear your baby's mouth and nose of any fluids. Since they are not going through the vaginal canal, which naturally squeezes fluids out of their lungs, they may need some assistance getting fluids out. Then once their whole body is delivered, your doctor should hold your beautiful baby up so you can see him or her. Some care providers will first pass your baby to the nurse for a quick evaluation, and if your baby is healthy then you should be able to get skin to skin right away, which is really important. You and your baby will be monitored closely for complications after the surgery and during your recovery.

Getting skin to skin is critical, especially for a baby who is born via a cesarean. There are many benefits of skin to skin contact. Being skin to skin stabilizes your baby's heart rate, breathing, and temperature, and reduces stress in both you and your baby. It also increases your interactions with your baby and increases the likelihood and length of breastfeeding. You can talk to your doctor about how soon you can hold your baby after they are born and let them know that it is a priority for you. Most hospitals are supportive of skin to skin contact right away, but definitely bring it up with your care provider well before your baby is born to find out how skin to skin contact works with a cesarean delivery.

Even with a cesarean you can still potentially delay clamping of the umbilical cord, have your placenta encapsulated, or bank cord blood. These topics are covered in detail in chapter 11. Work out the details of the timing of the cord clamping with your care provider beforehand. Regardless of what you choose to do with cord clamping, blood banking, or placenta encapsulation, the placenta will need to be removed from your uterus, you could feel some tugging while this is going on. Then the last thing your doctor will do is close up all of the incisions with sutures.

There are two options for how cesarean section uterine incisions can be closed, either with a single layer or a double layer of sutures. In the 1990's, the single-layer technique was touted as having fewer complications and became pretty widely accepted in the medical community, because short term it seemed like the single-layer technique was better. There have been questions raised about whether a single layer closure is linked to complications in the long term, specifically with a subsequent pregnancy. There have been links to higher rates of uterine rupture and placenta accreta, both of which can be life-threatening complications.

Ina May Gaskin, who is known as the authority on midwifery, has written a strong letter against the practice of suturing the uterine incision in one layer (Gaskin, Reprint of Email From Ina May Gaskin).

A study involving over 2,000 women from 1988-2000 concluded that a single-layer closure of the previous lower segment incision was the most influential factor and was associated with a 4-fold increase in the risk of uterine rupture compared with a double-layer closure (Bujold E. B. C., 2002). A study published in 2006 concluded that single-layer uterine closure might be more likely to result in uterine rupture. Of the 948 subjects in this study most had a double-layer closure and only 35 participants had a single-layer closure so that group was a much smaller sample size (Gyamfi C., 2006). A study published in 2010 with 288 participants concluded that prior single-layer closure carries more than twice the risk of uterine rupture compared with double-layer closure. Single-layer closure should be avoided in women who could contemplate future vaginal birth after cesarean delivery (Bujold E. G. M., 2010).

The International Cesarean Awareness Network (ICAN) is a non-profit organization aimed to reduce the current high cesarean rate and they published a paper that argues pretty strongly against the notion that a single-layer closure is associated with a higher risk of uterine rupture in a subsequent pregnancy and they argue that a single-layer closure has lower rates of complications following the surgery (Humphries, 2014). ICAN cites a study done with 768 women, of which 267 had a single-layer closure, and the study concluded that a single-layer uterine closure is associated with decreased blood loss, a shorter operating time, decreased cases of endometritis, and a shorter postoperative hospital stay. They go on to state that a single-layer closure is not associated with uterine rupture or other adverse outcomes in the subsequent pregnancy (Durnwald C., 2003).

If you are concerned about how your care provider will stitch up your incision from a cesarean section talk to them about it and ask them what their preferred procedure is and why. If you have any questions about long term risks if you have another baby then be sure to ask.

Like any other major surgery, C-sections carry risks and you will want to discuss these with your care provider in detail. Some of the risks include:

Endometritis, which is inflammation and infection of the membrane lining the uterus, and this can cause fever, foul smelling vaginal discharge and uterine pain.

You could have increased bleeding because you are likely to lose more blood with a C-section than with a vaginal birth.

You could have an adverse reaction to the anesthesia.

Blood clots can be a pretty serious risk and your chances of them are higher with a C-section than a vaginal delivery. Walking can help prevent blood clots and this is why your doctor will have you walking shortly after your surgery.

The incision could get infected.

Although it is rare, there is the possibility of an injury to nearby organs during the surgery, and this would require additional surgery to repair the injury.

There is an increased risk of complications in subsequent pregnancies, like a potential uterine rupture.

There are also some risks to your baby from a cesarean section. Problems breathing, like transient tachypnea, which is abnormally fast breathing during the first few days after birth, or respiratory distress syndrome which makes it difficult for your baby to breathe. Although it is rare, there is also the possibility of an accidental cut to your baby's skin during surgery.

There are a lot of reasons that you could be planning a scheduled C-Section for the birth of your baby. This is something you are going to be working with your doctor on and make sure that you are weighing all of your options, looking at all the scenarios, and doing what is best for you and your baby. Cesarean sections can be a lifesaving procedure, and there are times when it is safer to deliver a baby via C-section, and in those cases, we are very lucky to have that option available to us.

Some health conditions like heart disease, diabetes, high blood pressure or kidney disease could make a vaginal delivery very stressful to your body and your doctor may suggest that a C-section is a better option. If you have an infection that could be passed to your baby during a vaginal birth, like herpes or HIV, a C-section could prevent your baby from becoming infected. A C-section may also be needed if you have a mechanical obstruction like a large fibroid obstructing the birth canal, a severely displaced pelvic fracture, or if your baby has severe hydrocephalus, which is a condition that can cause their head to be unusually large. Your baby could have an illness or a congenital condition, like open neural tube defects, which could make a vaginal birth stressful for your little one. A C-section can be planned if your baby has a condition called macrosomia, which is a big word for having a large baby. Sometimes care providers will be concerned that a large baby will not be able to safely travel through the birth canal.

If your baby is in an abnormal position a C-section may be recommended. This could be if their feet or bottom enters the birth canal first, which is breech, or if your baby is positioned side or shoulder first, which is transverse. In cases of twins it is pretty common for one baby to be head down, and the other to be breech. Often if the first baby is head down and can be delivered vaginally, your doctor will deliver the second baby vaginally, even if they are breech. If you are expecting twins, find out what your care provider's policy is.

A C-section could be planned if there is a problem with your placenta. This could happen if have placenta previa, where your placenta covers the opening of your cervix. If you had some other kind of invasive uterine surgery, like a myomectomy, which is the surgical removal of fibroids you could have a planned C-section. Also if you have already had a previous C-section and are not considering a VBAC.

Other complications like preeclampsia, which is pregnancy-induced high blood pressure, or eclampsia, which is a very rare progression of preeclampsia, your practitioner might suggest a cesarean to protect both of you and your baby.

Obesity significantly increases your chance of needing a C-section. This is partially due to other risk factors that often accompany obesity, and partially because obese women tend to have longer labors, which can increase your risk of having a C-section.

The last reason you may have a planned C-section is just because that is how you want to deliver your baby, and an elective C-section is an option. Doctors generally will not do an elective C-section prior to 39 weeks. You know those last few weeks are really critical for lung development. If this is something you are considering, as with any intervention, you definitely want to talk it over with your care provider, do your research, and weigh the pros and cons to make sure you are making the best decision for you and your baby.

There are quite a few reasons that you could have an unplanned or an emergency C-section. Don't let this list freak you out. The more you plan and prepare for the birth experience you want, the more you will minimize the chances of a cesarean section. Even if the last thing in the world you want is a C-section getting educated about what is involved and what your options are will be beneficial. Talk to your care provider about the possibility of a C-section and what their procedures are. Ask any questions you have, share any of your concerns, and your partner's concerns. If you do this beforehand, and something doesn't go as planned, and you end up meeting your baby via cesarean you will be so much better off going into this knowing what to expect and knowing what your options are. In an emergency scenario, your doctor may not be able to fully explain the procedure and answer all of your questions. Over 25% of C-sections are with low-risk pregnancies (Osterman, 2014), a lot of these are women who went into labor planning not to have a C-section.

One big reason, and the most common reason, for an unplanned C-section is that your labor is not progressing. You should be well versed in the interventions, both artificial and natural, that can be applied in this case. There are some interventions that increase your risk for a cesarean section. Some other reasons for an unplanned C-section include:

Your baby's heart rate will be monitored during labor and if your doctor is concerned that your baby is not getting enough oxygen, they may suggest a C-section.

If there is a problem with the umbilical cord, which could happen if the umbilical cord slips through your cervix ahead of your baby, this is called a prolapsed umbilical cord. If the cord is compressed by the uterus during contractions or is compressed as your baby comes through, and is cutting off the oxygen supply to your baby, this could create the need for a C-section.

In the case of a placental abruption, which means your placenta starts to separate from your uterine wall, an emergency C-section is done. A placental abruption can compromise your baby's oxygen supply, and that is why it is considered an emergency.

You can see that there are some things that can be out of your control and create the need for a cesarean section. Even if you are planning the most natural birth possible, it is a good idea to know about C-sections just as some emergency preparation if it were to come up.

For more information on cesarean sections you can listen to episode 39 of the Pregnancy Podcast at PregnancyPodcast.com/episode39.

Vaginal Birth After Cesarean (VBAC)

VBAC stands for vaginal birth after cesarean. In the past it was assumed once you had one cesarean section, every subsequent birth would also need to be via cesarean. A VBAC is not recommended if you had a uterine rupture during a previous pregnancy or if you had a classical incision in a C-section. A classical incision is a vertical incision in the upper part of your uterus and this carries a higher risk of uterine rupture than the more commonly used low transverse uterine incision. A uterine rupture can occur when your uterus tears along a scar from a previous C-section, and this requires an emergency C-section.

Today VBAC is becoming more popular. The majority of women who have had a cesarean are a candidate for a VBAC. Of women who plan for a VBAC, about 60-80% are successful (American Congress of Obstetricians and Gynecologists, 2010).

If you are planning a VBAC the first and most important step is to work with a doctor or midwife who is supportive of your decision and make sure they are 100% on board with your birth plan. Also, make sure to discuss your plan B in the event a cesarean becomes necessary. There are a few things you can do to increase your chances of a successful vaginal delivery.

If you are planning a VBAC take into consideration any interventions that could increase your risk for a cesarean. Interventions are discussed in detail in Chapter 8. A study of over 6,000 women attempting a VBAC did find that induction of labor before 40 weeks in women with one prior cesarean delivery is associated with an increased risk of failed VBAC, and required a cesarean delivery (Lappen J.R., 2015).

To increase your success of having a VBAC you want to stack the odds in your favor as much as possible. The more things you can do to decrease your risk of having a C-section, the better. First you definitely want to be working with a doctor or midwife who is supportive of VBACs. There is some research that shows inducing labor increases the risk of a failed cesarean, so the preference would be to go into labor naturally without an induction. Getting a doula could be a huge asset for you during your labor and birth as studies show having a doula decreases your risk of having a cesarean (Hodnett E.D., 2012).

Chapter 9: Natural Birth

Natural birth is defined as childbirth without routine medical interventions, particularly anesthesia.

Let's take a look at what the natural birth process looks like from beginning to end, without interventions. Our understanding of this process, the hormones involved, and how they impact labor and birth is constantly improving. We do not know exactly how everything works but our overall understanding of the uninterrupted birth process may help explain why some moms choose a natural birth.

As your baby and your body get ready to go into labor your placenta triggers an increase in prostaglandins that soften the cervix to prepare it for effacing and dilating. Your levels of estrogen rise and the levels of progesterone decrease which makes the uterus more sensitive to oxytocin. During labor and birth oxytocin is the driving force of your contractions. In cases of a labor with interventions, Pitocin is commonly used to both start labor and progress labor, and this is a synthetic version of oxytocin. Your labor will progress best in an environment where you feel safe and relaxed. In the wild most animals retreat to a quiet safe place to give birth. If there is any sign of danger their bodies will literally halt the birth so they can react to the threat and find safety. Humans operate the same way. Part of having a natural birth is being in an environment where you feel safe and supported to allow your body to do what it needs to do. Oxytocin is the hormone primarily responsible for causing your contractions, and the levels of oxytocin will be highest when you are in a safe environment. It is really this symphony of everything working together in sync that starts your labor naturally, when both you and your baby are ready.

As part of the natural labor process, in the first stage of labor when your cervix is dilating and effacing, your body produces a hormone called beta-endorphin. Beta-endorphin is a stress hormone, and it is released under conditions of duress. This hormone acts as an opiate or painkiller. It also suppresses the immune system, which is thought to be important in preventing your immune system from acting against your baby, who has different genetic make-up from you. When you are in labor and high levels of beta-endorphin are released this is going to reduce the levels of oxytocin being released, which can slow down your contractions. While this may seem counterproductive to birth, this keeps labor at a pace where you are able to experience the positive effects and relief from beta endorphins, and at a pace where your body can handle the stress. Beta-endorphin is similar to morphine. This applies to more than the pain relief aspect of it, and beta endorphins induce feelings of pleasure and euphoria. The high levels being released during birth help you enter an altered state of consciousness. This might sound a little out there, and what this basically means is that you are on a high, similar to being high on a drug, but without any of the negative side effects. You will sometimes hear birth educators or practitioners talk about a birthing mother being in labor land. This is used to describe this sort of meditative state where you are zoned out of what is going on around you and focused on what is going on internally with your baby and your body.

At the end of the first stage of labor your cervix is fully dilated at 10 centimeters and you enter the transition phase which is taking you into the second, or pushing stage of labor. This is where your fight-or-flight hormones come in, which are classified as catecholamines. These include adrenaline, also called epinephrine, and noradrenaline, also known as norepinephrine. These hormones are secreted from your adrenal gland in response to stress, and they get your body ready for a fight-or-flight response. While these hormones can slow things down a bit in the first stage of labor, they act differently in the second stage just before your baby is born. Right before the moment of birth there is a sudden increase in catecholamines, especially noradrenaline, and this works with oxytocin, which activates the fetal ejection reflex. Stereotypically when this happens you are going to get a sudden rush of energy, you will be upright and alert, your mouth will be dry, and your breathing will be shallow. You could express fear, anger, or excitement, and the rush of these fight or flight hormones is going to cause several very strong contractions, which are designed to birth your baby quickly and easily. These hormones will also act to help your baby during birth by protecting them against the effects of hypoxia, which is a lack of oxygen, because when your uterus contracts oxygen flow is temporarily restricted. After the birth, your levels of catecholamines drop sharply which will help your body release more oxytocin.

Once your baby is born you will immediately get skin to skin. Oxytocin is continuing to be released which is going to continue contractions, which will be much milder than the ones you experienced during birth. The purpose of the continued contractions is to push the placenta out of your uterus, close off the blood vessels that were attached to it, and start shrinking your uterus. This process is important to prevent postpartum hemorrhage, which is heavy bleeding and can be a serious complication.

All of the hormones you are producing during birth are also being transferred to your baby. Immediately following birth both you and your baby are going to have really high levels of oxytocin and this is going to help promote bonding. The fight or flight hormones are going to make your baby alert for their first contact with you. The skin to skin contact after birth is going to soothe your little one and help to lower those levels of adrenaline and noradrenaline.

One of the first things that happens naturally after birth is that your baby instinctively wants to latch on to breastfeed. If a newborn is placed on your abdomen after birth they will use all of their senses (sight, touch, taste, smell, and sound) to instinctively crawl up to your breast and latch on. Babies come pre wired to breastfeed and birth hormones have a lot to do with the process of your body producing milk and the breastfeeding relationship. The hormone most associated with breastfeeding is prolactin, and it is also known as the mothering hormone. Throughout your pregnancy you be producing higher than normal levels of prolactin but production of milk is inhibited until the third stage of labor when you birth the placenta. Your level of prolactin decreases during labor, increases at the end of your labor, then peaks at birth. This hormone is going to help with breastfeeding, not just by physically helping you to produce milk, but it also fosters nurturance from you to your baby and that will overall help your breastfeeding relationship. Another factor that will help breastfeeding is a peak in your levels of beta-endorphin about 20 minutes after birth; this also ends up in your breast milk and fosters some dependency between you and your baby. Oxytocin also plays a part to help promote the letdown reflex, which is the reflex that causes milk, or initially colostrum, to be released, and this is going to help signal your body to produce milk.

You can see that labor and birth is a really complex process with a lot of moving parts. Although we are constantly improving our understanding of how everything works with a natural labor, we do not fully know the effects of everything going on.

There are some expecting moms who are at a high-risk and their doctor or midwife would not recommend a natural birth or they may recommend some interventions or procedures. You will need to be working with your care provider to decide which course of action is going to be the best one for you to take and weigh the benefits and risks of your specific situation. The bottom line is that you have choices. You do not have to make a choice between having your baby in a bathtub at home or in a hospital with a C-section. Your birth is not a black and white choice between two opposing options. You have an infinite number of options and there are a lot of shades of grey where you can combine the tools, techniques, and procedures you think will be best for you and your baby and really craft the birth experience you want.

For more information on natural birth you can listen to episode 40 of the Pregnancy Podcast at PregnancyPodcast.com/episode40.

Chapter 10: Water Birth

There are legends of women in different cultures laboring in water dating back quite a ways but there isn't documentation of anyone actually giving birth in water until 1803 in France. Then it wasn't until the 1980's that the popularity of water births began growing in Western cultures, and today it is becoming increasingly popular. Proponents of water birth claim that it is beneficial in management of discomfort from contractions, that it promotes relaxation, and that it eases stress for your baby during birth. Critics of the practice raise concerns about the safety of water birth, risks associated with respiratory issues for your baby, and the risk of infection for both you and your baby.

Water birth may be an option for you if you are planning a natural labor and are considered low-risk. You will need to be planning on having your baby at a venue that accommodates water birth, with a care provider who is supportive of the practice, and who has experience attending water births. While more hospitals are beginning to offer this as an option, the majority of water births are taking place in homes or at birth centers, under the care of a midwife.

During a water birth you are partially immersed in a tub of warm water. The temperature of the water is about body temperature. Generally the tub is larger than a standard bathtub and is either a built-in tub or a portable inflatable pool. You will be naked from the waist down in a tub during labor. Some women choose to wear a sports bra and some women prefer not to wear anything, ultimately whatever you are most comfortable in. Your partner may be able to join you in the tub if that would assist you. Even if you are not sure if you will want your partner in the tub, they should have swimwear on hand just in case.

Immersion in water could be helpful in the first stage of labor even if you are not planning to birth your baby, or go through the second stage of labor in the tub. In a tub of warm water you are free to move around in different positions and may find some relief from the buoyancy of water. If you do choose to have an underwater birth and be immersed in water for the second stage of labor you should know that it is common for babies born in water to take a little bit longer to get their color.

Your labor is going to progress best when you are comfortable. Your needs and the positions you choose will evolve as your labor progresses. It is possible you find being in a tub wonderful in the beginning and at some point decide you prefer to be on dry land. Give yourself some wiggle room to change your plans if needed and if at any point a tub isn't working for you, get out and try something else. You can always get back in.

One of the most common questions about water birth is whether your baby could drown under water. The first thing you should know is that your baby's oxygen supply is coming through the umbilical cord. Your baby's oxygen supply is monitored by their heart rate, which would slow down in the event they were not getting enough oxygen from the placenta. Your care provider will be intermittently monitoring your baby's heart rate with a hand held waterproof Doppler. There is a complex chain reaction that takes place once a baby is born that initiates their first breath of air. Once your baby is born you or your care provider would be gently lifting them out of the water where they would take their first breath of air, and you wouldn't leave them in the water for any extended period of time.

A review of 12 trials, including over 3,200 women found that being immersed in water for the first stage of labor was associated with a significant reduction in the rates of epidural or other types of anesthesia and the first stage of labor was about a half of an hour shorter. There was no difference in the rates of assisted vaginal deliveries, cesarean sections, use of Pitocin, perineal trauma, or maternal infection. There were also no differences in neonatal outcomes for Apgar scores of less than seven at five minutes, neonatal unit admissions, or neonatal infection rates. Of the three trials that compared water immersion during the second stage with no immersion, one trial showed a significantly higher level of satisfaction with the birth experience. This review did note that a lack of data for some comparisons prevented robust conclusions and further research is needed (Cluett, 2009). Another study found that water births had shorter second and third stages of labor compared to vaginal deliveries on dry land, both with and without an epidural (Mollamahmutoğlu L., 2012).

An Italian study of 2,625 water births found shorter labor duration, a net reduction in episiotomy rate, and a marked drop in requests for pain relievers. The study mentions that during the birth of the baby, fecal matter is released into the birth pool water, contaminating it with microorganisms. Despite this, water birthing was found to be safe for the neonate and did not carry a higher risk of neonatal infection when compared with conventional vaginal delivery (Thöni A., 2010).

As is the case with so many pregnancy and birth procedures there is no perfectly controlled study that gives us a solid answer as to whether water birth is safe and effective. Two major authorities on pregnancy and birth, the American Academy of Pediatrics and the American Congress of Obstetricians and Gynecologists both agree on the official opinion issued on water births. Both organizations state that immersion in water during the first stage of labor may be associated with decreased pain or use of anesthesia and decreased duration of labor. They go on to state there is no evidence that immersion in water during the first stage of labor otherwise improves perinatal outcomes, and it should not prevent or inhibit other elements of care. The safety and efficacy of immersion in water during the second stage of labor have not been established, and immersion in water during the second stage of labor has not been associated with maternal or fetal benefit. Given these facts and case reports of rare but serious adverse effects in the newborn, the practice of immersion in the second stage of labor (underwater delivery) should be considered an experimental procedure that only should be performed within the context of an appropriately designed clinical trial with informed consent (American Academy of Pediatrics, 2014) (American Congress of Obstetricians and Gynecologists & The American Academy of Pediatrics, 2014).

The American College of Nurse Midwives has issued an official statement in support of water birth and states that labor and birth in water can be safely offered to women with uncomplicated pregnancies and should be made available by qualified maternity care providers. Labor and birth in water may be particularly useful for women who prefer physiological childbirth and wish to avoid use of pharmacological pain relief methods (American College of Nurse Midwives, 2014).

If you are interested in a water birth you will want to discuss your options with your care provider and make sure you are a good candidate given the specifics of your pregnancy and any possible risk factors. If water birth is not an option, because your care provider has concerns, or the policy of the hospital does not allow it, you may still be able to take advantage of some of the therapeutic aspects of water. You can take a warm bath in the early stages of labor at home. Once you are in labor at the hospital a shower may be soothing. You may even be able to take a plastic chair in the shower and sit on it backwards to get the shower on your back, which could be helpful and relaxing.

For more information on water birth you can listen to episode 45 of the Pregnancy Podcast at PregnancyPodcast.com/episode45.

Chapter 11: The Placenta and Umbilical Cord

When an egg is fertilized and the egg implants into your uterine wall the placenta starts forming. The placenta is an organ with a highly specialized purpose, and that is to support the normal growth and development of your baby. Oxygen and nutrients are transferred from you to your baby. Carbon dioxide and other waste products are transferred from your baby through the placenta and to your blood supply. Beginning around week 20 of your pregnancy, antibodies pass through the placenta to help protect your baby in utero. The antibodies being passed to your little one will help protect them during the first few months of their life and are the building blocks for their immune system. You already know that hormones rule everything during your pregnancy; your placenta plays a big role in secreting hormones that are crucial for your baby. This includes hCG, commonly known as the pregnancy hormone. HCG controls a lot and is also the indicator that turns your pregnancy test positive. The placenta secretes estrogen and progesterone and a few other hormones that are essential for your baby's development and your body during your pregnancy. Lastly, your placenta acts as a reservoir of blood for your little one. You can see that the placenta is a pretty amazing organ, your baby would not be able to survive without it.

The placenta is attached on one side to your uterus, and is connected to your baby by the umbilical cord. The umbilical cord is your baby's lifeline. At birth this will be about 20 inches, or 50-70 centimeters long, and .75 inches or 2 centimeters in diameter. The cord contains the umbilical vein, and two umbilical arteries. The umbilical vein carries nutrient rich, oxygenated blood from the placenta to your baby and the umbilical arteries carry deoxygenated, nutrient-depleted blood from your baby to the placenta.

Delayed Cord Clamping

When your baby is born blood will continue to flow between the placenta and your baby through the umbilical cord for a few minutes following birth. The net blood volume transferred to your baby during this time is called a placental transfusion. This transfer can give your baby about a fifth of their blood volume at birth, and this may make a difference to their health. This additional supply of blood provides extra iron, which can help guard against anemia in the first year of life, and it is enriched with immunoglobulins and stem cells. Placental transfusion drains the blood left in the placenta, which may help the placenta separate from the womb and may reduce overall blood loss at birth for you.

At some point after your baby is born, a clamp is put on the umbilical cord and the cord is cut. Once the cord is clamped, no blood is flowing so the timing between clamping it and cutting it is insignificant and usually cutting is done immediately after clamping it. The umbilical cord has no nerve endings so it is painless and neither you nor your little one will feel anything when this happens. The big question is when to do this. Do you clamp and cut the cord immediately or wait 3 minutes, or do you want to wait until the cord stops pulsating, which is closer to 10 minutes?

To cover all of your options there is something called a lotus birth, and this is where the cord is not cut at all. This means that your baby remains attached to the placenta until the cord naturally separates, and this usually happens somewhere between 3 and 10 days after birth. During this time the placenta is stored in a bag or container and must be carried around with your baby. The term lotus birth was coined in 1974 after Claire Lotus Day observed that chimpanzees do not sever the umbilical cord of their babies. This is not the most common practice but some mother's do it. If this is something you are considering you would definitely want to make sure that you are not exposing your little one to a risk of infection and talk to your care provider about the best way to minimize that risk.

The World Health Organization (WHO) recommends late cord clamping, which is performed approximately 1–3 minutes after birth. The WHO does not recommend early umbilical cord clamping, which would be less than one minute after birth, unless the there is an emergency where your baby needs to be moved immediately (World Health Organization, 2014).

The American Congress of Obstetricians and Gynecologists (ACOG) notes a study that found full term infants receive a transfer of approximately 80 ml of blood from the placenta in the first minute, and a total of 100 ml within three minutes. ACOG notes that systematic reviews of other studies have suggested that clamping the umbilical cord in all births should be delayed for at least 30–

60 seconds. The reasoning behind the recommendation to delay is based on the benefits including; increased blood volume, reduced need for blood transfusion, decreased incidence of intracranial hemorrhage in preterm infants, this is bleeding in the skull, and decreased frequency of iron deficiency anemia in term infants. In addition, a longer duration of placental transfusion after birth may be beneficial because this blood is enriched with immunoglobulins and stem cells, which provide the potential for improved organ repair and rebuilding after injury from disorders caused by preterm birth (American Congress of Obstetricians and Gynecologists Committee on Obstetric Practice, 2012).

Clearly there is a lot of evidence to support delayed clamping. How did the practice of clamping the cord immediately after birth ever start in the first place? This became pretty standard practice in the 1960's because it was thought to reduce the likelihood of postpartum maternal hemorrhage. The key word here is thought. Although more research needs to be done to know the effect of delayed cord clamping on maternal outcomes, immediate clamping does not reduce hemorrhaging. A review of 15 randomized trials involving a total of 3,911 women and infant pairs showed no significant difference in postpartum hemorrhage rates when early and late cord clamping (generally between one and three minutes) were compared. There were, however, some potentially important advantages of delayed cord clamping in healthy term infants, such as higher birth weight, early hemoglobin concentration, and increased iron reserves up to six months after birth. The study notes that these benefits need to be balanced against a small additional risk of jaundice in newborns, which requires phototherapy (McDonald S.J., 2013).

The main instance where immediate clamping would be necessary is in an emergency when you or your baby are in danger. As long as you and baby are doing well after birth, your care provider may delay clamping the cord.

Delayed cord clamping is not just for mothers who are having vaginal births with full term babies. This practice can still be applied if you are having a C-section or if your baby is premature.

There is still a transfer of blood that takes place after a cesarean birth and delayed cord clamping can still be beneficial. An approach your care provider may employ if you are having a C-section is to milk the umbilical cord. This is exactly what it sounds like, the cord is squeezed from the placenta towards the baby to help transfer blood between the two. In a C-section where time and speed are a concern, milking the cord may allow more of a transfer of blood.

Delayed clamping can be even more critical in a premature baby. There is a review of 15 randomized controlled trials with 738 babies born prematurely between 24 and 36 weeks' gestation by cesarean section or vaginal birth. These studies compared babies where the cord was clamped within a few seconds of the birth with those whose cords were clamped after a delay of at least 30 seconds. The maximum delay in cord clamping was 3 minutes. Providing babies with additional blood through delayed cord clamping or milking the cord before clamping helped the babies to adjust to their new surroundings. Fewer babies needed transfusions for anemia, the risk of bleeding in the brain (intraventricular hemorrhage) wa reduced, and the risk of a severe infection in the bowel (necrotizing enterocolitis) was reduced. Further studies are needed comparing the two methods of milking the cord or allowing it to transfer blood on its own, to deliver placental blood to babies to see which has the most benefit (Rabe H., 2012).

There is clear evidence that delaying cord clamping can be beneficial to both you and your baby. If this is something you want to do, the first thing is to ask your doctor or midwife what their practice or policy is. If they have a policy of clamping at one minute but you want to wait three minutes you need to make sure your wishes are known. Perhaps you are comfortable with your care provider clamping it at one minute. Or some women prefer to wait until the cord stops pulsating on its own and this usually is closer to 10 minutes.

For more information on delayed cord clamping you can listen to episode 26 of the Pregnancy Podcast at PregnancyPodcast.com/episode26.

Placenta Encapsulation

After the birth of your little boy or girl is the third stage of labor, and this stage involves the placenta detaching from your uterine wall and it will come out the same way your baby did. Once your baby is born should the placenta be discarded or could it be useful in helping you adapt and thrive in the postpartum period? Consumption of placenta by a mom after birth has been a taboo subject and has been gaining popularity in recent years. The thought of eating your placenta might gross you out at first but once you hear about some of the amazing benefits women claim it has you might be willing to consider it.

Human placentophagy is the technical term for eating your placenta. This can be either raw or altered by cooking, drying, or steeping it in liquid.

The list of potential benefits of placentophagy is pretty impressive and includes replenishing depleted iron, increasing energy, lessening the amount of postnatal bleeding, increasing milk production, balancing out hormones, and helping your uterus return to its pre-pregnancy state.

One of the biggest reported benefits of this list is balancing out hormones, which theoretically should help with the baby blues and/or postpartum depression. You have major drops in hormone levels following birth. If you have made it through your first trimester you know firsthand how hormones can make your moods swing all over the place and make you an emotional mess. Combine this with sleep deprivation, the physical stress after having a baby, your body healing, possibly dealing with breastfeeding challenges, and the stress of taking care of a newborn and you have the perfect storm to be bummed out after having your little one. The postpartum period is quite an adjustment as you are navigating being a new parent and your body is healing. If it is possible that consuming your placenta in some way could help you adjust it is definitely worth looking into.

There is no perfect placebo controlled study to give us black and white benefits or risks of consuming your placenta. Without a study showing a large group of women who ate their placenta, compared to a group who was given a placebo, the only evidence we have is anecdotal. The evidence we do have access to is a growing number of women who will rave on and on about how their experience with placenta encapsulation or eating their placenta raw was amazing. Just as no studies exist to prove any of the benefits, there are no studies that show that there is zero risk in consuming an organ that has acted as a filter to absorb and protect your developing baby from toxins and pollutants. Most of the time any conversation about placenta encapsulation is dominated with stories of how amazing it is, and many women feel it was an excellent choice. There has been some concern raised about the safety of ingesting your placenta.

If you really want to dig into the science side of this debate a computerized search of all of the big scientific journals from 1950 to 2014 for anything published in the scientific or medical community of placentophagy summarizes the findings of a total of 49 articles. The findings noted that overall the health benefits and risks of placentophagy require further investigation. As to risks, the placenta is not sterile and one function of the placenta is to protect the fetus from harmful exposure to substances. As a consequence, elements including selenium, cadmium, mercury, and lead, as well as bacteria have been identified in post-term placental tissues. There have been some studies on animals, such as rats, consuming placenta immediately after birth, but overall the results are inconclusive. From a scientific standpoint, more research is needed to determine whether benefits can be replicated in other populations with sound research methodology (Coyle C., 2014).

One resource, often cited as evidence of the benefits of placenta encapsulation, was a survey done by UNLV researchers who surveyed 189 women who ate their placenta, most of them in capsules. Overall, 96% of the women said they had a "positive" or "very positive" experience consuming their placenta, and 98% said they would do it again. About 57% of women in UNLV's study reported no negative effects from ingesting placenta. The most commonly reported negative experience revolved around the pill's taste and the "ick" factor of consuming placenta. As reported by the participants in the survey, the top positive effects were improved mood, increased energy, and improved lactation. The top negative side effects were unpleasant burping, headaches, and an unappealing taste or smell (Takahashi, 2013).

One recurring theme is the possibility that consuming placenta has positive effects due to the placebo effect. Obviously the reason anyone would encapsulate their placenta is because they perceive multiple postpartum health benefits. These are benefits drawn from the media, friends, family, doulas, midwives, and even doctors.

It would be easy to assume you can do whatever you want with your placenta, but that may not be the case. You need to check with your state and the hospital or birth center where you are planning to have your baby to make sure that you can remove your placenta. This shouldn't be an issue at most birth centers and it is becoming more and more common for hospitals to allow you to take your placenta home, or have someone else take it to prepare it. Some hospitals label the placenta as medical waste and deem it hazardous to release it to a patient to take home. This may be partly for liability reasons.

If you want your placenta after birth, check the policies of your care provider, talk to your doctor or midwife, and make sure it is an option.

There are many different ways that you could consume your placenta. Since the placenta is an organ, it should be treated just the same way meat would as far as safety goes. If you are planning to eat it raw it should be stored in the fridge and consumed within 3 days. You can also freeze it for up to six months. The most common way of eating your placenta raw is to put it in a smoothie. Another option is to cook it. A quick Google search will bring up recipes covering everything from lasagna to pizza and sandwiches. People get pretty creative with placenta recipes. Some moms prefer the raw method to cooking or drying the placenta because they believe that nutrients are lost during the steaming or cooking process. If all of this sounds off putting to you there is another option, which is much easier for many women to stomach, and that is placenta encapsulation. This is the most common, and perhaps the most socially accepted, method used.

Once your placenta is out, it should be refrigerated until it is treated and processed to be encapsulated. Typically, the person who is taking care of the encapsulation for you will pick up your placenta and the first step in the process is to drain and clean it. The next step will vary depending on the method being used to encapsulate your placenta. According to the traditional Chinese medicine method, it is steamed with herbs. Traditionally this includes lemongrass, ginger, and spicy green pepper. The other option is the raw method, which skips the step of steaming it with herbs. If you are into raw foods and eat a raw food diet, this option may be more aligned with your lifestyle. The next steps are the same regardless of the method being used. The placenta is sliced very thinly and put in a dehydrator. Once the placenta is dehydrated, it is ground up and put into gel capsules. There are different types of gel capsules and if it is important for you to have vegetarian or vegan capsules, or if you want to know your options on this be sure to ask about it. This entire process takes between 1-3 days and once the capsules are done they are delivered to you and you can start taking them right away. You will want to store them in a cool dry place and probably take a few capsules a couple of times a day. Depending on your total supply, you should have pills for about a month, and you would want to take these within 6-12 months max. There is no standard on dosage. Talk with your care provider and the person who will be encapsulating your placenta to figure out what will be best for you.

It is possible to DIY placenta encapsulation if you want to get really hands on. If you are considering this keep in mind that you will probably have your hands pretty full, especially in the first few days. Most moms who choose to have their placenta encapsulated will outsource it to a doula or midwife who specializes in the process.

The last option available to you is to have a tincture made from your placenta. This is a good option to stretch out the length of time you can use it. A small portion of your placenta is added to over 100 proof alcohol and ferments for 6 weeks. There are women who do this and save it to take later as a mood stabilizer during their menstrual cycle to help with PMS or even much later in life when they are going through menopause. We aren't going to get into the possible pros and cons of taking this after your postpartum period but if this is something you may want to consider talk to your encapsulation specialist about it.

There are several organizations that offer a training program and a certification for placenta encapsulation. This includes the Association for Placenta Preparation Arts, PlacentaBenefits.info (PBi), and the International Placenta and Postpartum Association. There is no nationally accredited certification program. If you are looking into multiple providers of this service it may be worth it to ask if they have any type of certification and how many clients they have done it for. If placenta encapsulation is something you are considering look into it and talk to some specialists, or even ask around to find out if anyone you know has an experience with it. If you aren't sure whether or not you want to do this contact a placenta specialist and ask them any questions you have to make a decision about it.

For more information on placenta encapsulation you can listen to episode 28 of the Pregnancy Podcast at PregnancyPodcast.com/episode28.

Cord Blood Banking

Cord blood contains hematopoietic stem cells that can form red blood cells, white blood cells, and platelets. The ability to differentiate into these types of blood cells can make cord blood helpful in treating blood and immune system related genetic diseases, cancers, and blood disorders. You can collect a sample of cord blood right after your baby is born and then have it stored in a cord blood bank to potentially be used at a later date.

The first clinically documented use of cord blood stem cells was in the successful treatment of a six-year-old boy afflicted by Fanconi anemia in 1988. Since then, cord blood has become increasingly recognized as a source of stem cells that could be used in stem cell therapy. There is a fairly long list of illnesses (nearly 80) that may be treated with cord blood. This includes many types of cancers, bone marrow failure syndromes, blood disorders, metabolic disorders, immunodeficiency, and some other diseases like osteoporosis. Take note that these are not common, and your little one has a very small chance of having any of these illnesses. If you have a family history of any disorders or diseases it may be worth talk to your care provider about whether cord blood banking could potentially help treat the condition, in the event your baby, or someone else in your family has it.

While cord blood banking is often marketed as biological insurance, you cannot assume that your baby would be able to use their own cord blood. Often, children who develop an immunological disorder are unable to use their own cord blood for transplant because their blood also contains the same genetic defect. This is common with leukemia, which is a cancer and the largest use of cord blood stem cells.

A cord blood bank is a facility that stores umbilical cord blood for future use. When you store your baby's cord blood at a private bank it is stored solely for the potential use by your baby or your family. There are no accurate estimates of the likelihood of children who need their own stored cord blood stem cells in the future. Private banks do charge a fairly high fee, typically around $2,000 USD for the collection, and around $200 USD a year for storage. This could vary from one company to the next, but this is a good ballpark figure of what you can expect to spend. There is some controversy in the medical community about private for-profit cord blood banks, and whether physicians, employees, and consultants of private banks have potential conflicts of interest in recruiting patients because of their own financial gain.

If you choose to store your baby's cord blood at a public bank, it works very much like a blood bank, and you don't own the cord blood donated. Public cord blood banks accept donations from anyone, they discard donations that don't meet their quality control standards, and they use national registries to find recipients for their samples. Some of the public cord blood banks are programs funded by the National Heart Lung and Blood Institute, the National Marrow Donor Program, the American Red Cross, or academic programs based in not-for-profit organizations. Samples sent to a public bank are tested for chromosomal abnormalities and infectious diseases and if abnormalities are identified, you will be notified. It is important to note that cord blood banked in a public program may not be accessible for future private use. It is also a possibility your donation could be life saving for someone else. Public banks generally do not charge any fees.

Since patients who need cord blood frequently need more cells than a single collection would have provided, public banks frequently combine multiple samples together when preparing the treatment for a single patient. If someone needs a cord blood transplant as an adult, they will need an even larger sample because their body is larger than a child. Many cord blood samples may be too small to be used for transplantation because they don't contain enough stem cells. A private bank will store a sample, even if it is too small, because you are paying them for that service. Public banks will discard any samples that do not collect enough usable cells. The percentage of public bank donations discarded as medical waste is often cited to be between 60% and 80%. Some of this is due to contamination that can occur during collection or complications arising from shipping, but this is mostly due to the collection not collecting enough usable cells.

You can see a few reasons why public cord banks are more widely accepted in the medical community. Overall the attitude is that private banks have lower quality control and lower medical usefulness of using a patient's own cord blood. Matches are almost always likely to be better in a public bank rather than a private bank. The American Academy of Pediatrics states that cord blood donation should be discouraged when cord blood stored in a bank is to be directed for later personal or family use, because most conditions that might be helped by cord blood stem cells already exist in the infant's cord blood. The cord blood stem cell collection program should not alter routine practice for the timing of umbilical cord clamping (American Academy of Pediatrics, 2007). The American Medical Association recommends that private banking should be considered in the unusual circumstance when there exists a family predisposition to a condition in which umbilical cord stem cells are therapeutically indicated. However, because of its cost, limited likelihood of use, and inaccessibility to others, private banking should not be recommended to low-risk families (American Medical Association, 2008).

If you choose to use a cord blood bank, the way most companies work is you sign up with them, complete some paperwork, and they send you a collection kit, which you take with you to the delivery. Cord blood collection happens after the umbilical cord has been cut and your care provider or a nurse collects the sample from the end of the cord that was attached to your baby. This is usually done within ten minutes of giving birth. After the collection a medical courier picks up the cord blood and delivers it to the cord blood bank.

An adequate cord blood collection requires at least 50-75 ml in order to ensure that there will be enough cells to be used for transplantation. Keep in mind about 80 ml of blood is transferred from the placenta to your baby in the first minute after birth, and this amount increases to about 100 ml within three minutes. You can see that there could be a conflict if you want to both delay cord clamping and bank cord blood. The placenta contains approximately 200 ml of blood, although that doesn't mean that exactly 200 ml of blood could be extracted from it.

The short answer is that delaying clamping and cord blood banking are not mutually exclusive, you can potentially do both, but the delay should be brief. According to the American Academy of Pediatrics, if you are banking cord blood, you can delay cord clamping, as long as the delay is brief – no more than a minute or two (American Academy of Pediatrics, 2007). The American Congress of Obstetricians and Gynecologists (ACOG) states that it is possible to delay clamping and collect enough cord blood to bank it. ACOG states that only about 50 milliliters (ml) of blood is necessary for cord blood storage, which is just a portion of the approximately 200 ml of blood contained in the placenta and umbilical cord. If you choose to delay the cord clamping by 1 minute, around 80 ml of this blood is transferred to your baby, leaving more than enough to be stored in a cord blood bank. Even if you delay clamping by 3 minutes, only around 100 ml will have gone into the baby. They recommend that you probably don't want to wait to clamp the umbilical cord for much longer than 3 minutes to ensure you'll have enough for cord blood storage (American Congress of Obstetricians and Gynecologists, 2015; Australian Institute of Health and Welfare, 2013).

If you are considering cord blood banking, and want to delay cord clamping, you should talk to your doctor or midwife, since they will likely be the person actually taking the sample. Ask them for a specific time frame and for their opinion on delaying clamping and whether they feel that you can still get an adequate sample size after a delay of whatever the length of time is that you want to delay clamping and cutting your baby's cord.

For more information on cord blood banking you can listen to episode 27 of the Pregnancy Podcast at PregnancyPodcast.com/episode27.

The Third Stage of Labor

The third stage of labor starts after your baby is born and ends with birthing the placenta. Once your beautiful baby is born your uterus continues to contract and shrink, and your placenta will detach from your uterine wall. The blood vessels are then closed off and the placenta is pushed out.

The main complications that can arise during the third stage of labor are postpartum hemorrhage, a retained placenta, and uterine inversion.

Postpartum hemorrhage is the number one cause of maternal mortality. In general, postpartum hemorrhage occurs when a mother loses over 500 ml of blood in a vaginal birth or 1,000 ml of blood in a cesarean birth. These figures may vary between countries and there is no universal measurement. Care providers can only estimate the amount of blood lost, they cannot accurately measure it. Postpartum hemorrhage is more common in low-income countries where access to care is limited. Over the last few decades, rates of postpartum hemorrhage have been on the rise in developed countries and unfortunately researchers have not been able to pinpoint the cause of this.

A retained placenta occurs when the placenta does not detach from the uterine wall. The risks involved with this include hemorrhage and infection. The amount of time your care provider is comfortable waiting for your placenta to be delivered without interventions will vary, and can range from 30 minutes to 2 hours.

Uterine inversion occurs when the placenta does not detach from the uterine wall and as it is pushed out it draws the uterus with it, turning the organ inside out.

It is a high priority of your doctor or midwife to make sure that your third stage of labor goes smoothly, and the placenta is delivered without complications. You have two main choices when it comes to how to birth your placenta; expectant management or active management. Advocates of expectant management argue that the natural process your body goes through promotes normal separation and birth of the placenta and minimizes complications. Proponents of an active approach argue that that active management is quicker and results in fewer complications.

Expectant management, sometimes also called physiological, means that the cord is not clamped early, no medications are administered, and there is no pulling on the umbilical cord. Advocates of this method argue that any interference with the natural cascade of hormones that occurs immediately following birth has impacts on both you and your baby. In general, mothers who are planning a natural birth opt for expectant management, which is more in line with their ideology on birth.

Active management usually involves early cord clamping, administration of medication, and gently pulling the umbilical cord.

It is also possible to have a combination of these two methods, sometimes referred to as mixed management, where some but not all of the methods of active management are employed.

A review of seven studies involving over 8,000 women found that active management of the third stage reduced the risk of hemorrhage greater than 1000 ml at the time of birth, but adverse effects were identified. The review concluded that given the concerns about early cord clamping and the potential adverse effects of some medications, it is critical to look at the individual components of third stage management (Begley CM, 2015).

A look into the individual components of active management will give you a better idea of what methods you would like to use or avoid during the third stage of labor.

There is quite a bit of evidence to support delayed cord clamping and this topic is covered in depth in the beginning of this chapter.

The medications given during active management of the third stage of labor are classified as uterotonic agents. These drugs increase contractions and are given either orally, through an IV, or with a shot. There are four main types of uterotonics; oxytocin, carbetocin, ergot derivatives and prostaglandins. Oxytocin is your body's natural hormone to create contractions, and there are also synthetic versions of this. Carbetocin is available in the U.K. and Canada, but not in the United States. Ergot derivatives include Syntometrine, a combination of oxytocin and ergometrine. Prostaglandins include misoprostol, which is marketed under the brand name, Cytotec.

A review of six trials involving over 9,300 women compared Syntometrine, a combination of oxytocin and ergometrine, with Syntocinon, which is oxytocin only. The review found that the combination drug was associated with fewer instances of postpartum hemorrhage but had more side effects, notably vomiting, nausea and hypertension (McDonald SJ, 2004).

A review of 72 trials involving over 52,000 women examined the use of prostaglandins, specifically misoprostol, which is taken orally. When misoprostol was used compared to no other drugs it did lower the risk for postpartum hemorrhage and blood transfusions. Compared to other uterotonics, misoprostol had higher rates of severe postpartum hemorrhage and use of additional uterotonics, but fewer blood transfusions. The review also found that misoprostol is associated with significant increases in shivering and a temperature of 100.4° Fahrenheit, or 38° Celsius, compared with both a placebo and other uterotonics. Overall, misoprostol is not as effective as oxytocin, and it has more side effects (Tunçalp Ö, 2012). In areas where access to medical care is limited an oral medication, like misoprostol, may have more application.

A review of 20 trials involving over 10,800 women found that oxytocin reduced the rates of postpartum hemorrhage. When compared to ergot alkaloids, oxytocin was more effective and had fewer side effects. There was also no benefit found in combining oxytocin with ergometrine, the combination drug known as Syntometrine. There was no evidence suggesting that retained placentas were more common with use of oxytocin (Westhoff G, 2013).

If you are planning to have a uterotonic administered during the third stage of labor it may be helpful to discuss your options with your care provider and discuss the risks and benefits of the different medications available.

Your care provider can also use controlled cord traction, and apply traction to the cord by gently pulling it to assist in the delivery of the placenta. They may also put pressure on your uterus to help it contract. There is a method to this, and any care provider performing controlled cord traction should be skilled in the technique.

A review of three trials involving over 27,000 focused on controlled cord traction and found that there was no difference in the risk of blood loss over 1,000 ml but that it did reduce blood loss of more than 500 ml. There were no clear differences in use of additional uterotonics, blood transfusion, maternal death, operative procedures, nor maternal satisfaction (Hofmeyr GJ, 2015).

When you are figuring out what methods you want to use or avoid during the third stage of labor talk to your doctor or midwife and find out what their policy and recommendation is. From there you can discuss your options and any concerns to figure out what route you want to take.

For more information on the third stage of labor you can listen to episode 48 of the Pregnancy Podcast at PregnancyPodcast.com/episode48.

Chapter 12: Breastfeeding

Breastfeeding is arguably the best thing you can do for baby. There is no formula that comes close to mimicking breast milk. Your milk contains every vitamin, mineral, and nutritional element your baby needs. It contains living cells to inhibit the growth of bacteria and viruses. Babies who are breastfed are at a lower risk for ear infections, intestinal upsets, respiratory problems, allergies, dental problems, and their immune system will be stronger. Breastfeeding produces prolactin and oxytocin, which are hormones that foster a connection to your baby and help you recover from birth. The best way to get breastfeeding off to a great start is to be skin to skin with your baby.

For more information on breastfeeding you can listen to episode 10 of the Pregnancy Podcast at PregnancyPodcast.com/episode10.

To get tips on preparing for breastfeeding you can listen to episode 29 of the Pregnancy Podcast at PregnancyPodcast.com/episode29.

Colostrum

During your pregnancy your body starts producing colostrum. This first milk has immunological properties. Most importantly, colostrum contains high concentrations of secretory immunoglobulin A. This is an anti-infective agent that coats their intestines to protect against the passage of germs and foreign proteins that could create allergic sensitivities. Another ingredient in colostrum is pancreatic secretory trypsin inhibitor, which protects and repairs the infant's intestine. It may not seem like very much but at birth your baby's stomach is the size of a marble. Colostrum is nature's perfect food until your milk comes in.

Formula

Today most hospitals and care providers are extremely supportive of breastfeeding and will have a lactation consultant on staff that can come by for a visit after your baby is born. Take advantage of this resource to help you get off to a great start. If you do not want to supplement with formula do not hesitate to let your care provider know. If you are planning to supplement with formula from the start and you want to know what formula your baby will be getting ask your care provider what the hospital provides and you can always bring your own with you if things like organic or non GMO ingredients are important to you.

For more information on infant formula you can listen to episode 33 of the Pregnancy Podcast at PregnancyPodcast.com/episode33.

Pacifiers

Whether or not you choose to give your baby a pacifier is entirely up to you. While it may seem obvious to give your baby a pacifier, some parents choose not to do it. The only reason you would include anything about pacifiers in your birth plan is if you do not want to use them, in which case you may want to make sure the hospital or birth center does not give one to your baby.

There are both pros and cons to pacifiers and by understanding both sides you can decide whether giving your baby a pacifier is the right move for you. Pacifiers are designed to pacify your baby. At one point or another you have seen a mom give a fussy baby a pacifier, which can immediately calm them down. Babies start building their strong sucking reflex in the womb. This is needed for breastfeeding and nutrition but it also has a calming effect and many babies find it soothing.

Let's start with the pros. A crying baby can be stressful and it can be a challenge to run through a list of things to try and soothe them. Often, giving them a pacifier will instantly calm them down. A pacifier can also serve as a good distraction when you are visiting the pediatrician or want to do something your baby doesn't enjoy like clipping or filing their nails. A pacifier can be helpful in settling your baby to sleep. On a flight a pacifier may help your little one equalize their ears during air pressure changes during takeoff and landing. Giving your baby a pacifier may even decrease the risk of SIDS. You can see there are a lot of times when having a pacifier can be handy, and a lot of parents would consider them to be a necessity.

There are also cons to giving your baby a pacifier. Early pacifier use could interfere with breastfeeding. Your baby could become dependent on a pacifier, which could be troublesome if they need it to go to sleep, then wake up crying when it falls out of their mouth during the night. If your baby uses a pacifier it could increase their risk of middle ear infections. It is worth noting that the risk of middle ear infections is lowest in the first six months, which is also the time your baby will be most interested in a pacifier. If your baby ends up using a pacifier long term it could create dental issues with the development of their mouth and the alignment of their teeth.

Some practitioners refer to using a pacifier as nonnutritive sucking, as opposed to nutritive sucking while breastfeeding or drinking from a bottle. A review from the American Medical Association did not find pacifiers to be detrimental to breastfeeding outcomes but overall it did find that early use of pacifiers could be associated with decreased exclusive breastfeeding, and the duration of breastfeeding (O'Connor N.R., 2009). If you are breastfeeding, you can wait to offer a pacifier to your baby until breastfeeding is well established and they are at least 3 or 4 weeks old. The first few weeks are also very important to establishing your milk supply and the more often you are breastfeeding the better. Using a pacifier could substitute some times that you would be putting your baby to your breast to soothe them.

There is some evidence that pacifiers lower the risk of sudden infant death syndrome (SIDS). The American Academy of Pediatrics recommends parents consider offering a pacifier at naptime and bedtime. Although the mechanism is yet unclear, studies show a protective effect on the use of a pacifier and the instances of SIDS (American Academy of Pediatrics, 2011).

There are reasons to both offer your baby a pacifier and reasons not to use one. If you prefer not to use a pacifier or would like to wait to introduce one make sure your care provider and the venue where you are giving birth is aware of your preference.

Chapter 13: Procedures after birth

There are a lot of procedures that can happen to your baby shortly after birth. Whether these procedures occur and when depends on where you give birth and what you and your care provider have planned. While a number of procedures have become routine, that does not always mean that they are mandatory. You have options when it comes to what procedures are done on your baby and whether or not you choose to opt in, delay, or opt out of these.

Skin to Skin

No matter what type of birth you have, the most important thing is that you get skin to skin with your baby as soon as possible. Skin to skin means that your baby is not swaddled or clothed and their bare skin is placed belly down against your bare chest. A blanket is then put over you and your baby to keep both of you warm. The first hour after birth your baby will be pretty alert, enjoy every second with that little one. If you do choose to opt in to some procedures many of them can be performed while your baby is on your chest.

Kangaroo care is a term for skin to skin contact that was initially developed for preterm babies. Today, kangaroo care is practiced in many neonatal intensive care units around the world with successful results. The World Health Organization has developed a set of guidelines involving other recommendations, in addition to skin to skin contact, called Kangaroo Mother Care.

From an evolutionary perspective skin to skin contact was necessary for the survival of a newborn. According to mammalian neuroscience, intimate contact evokes neurobehavioral action needed to fulfill basic biological needs. This time may represent a psycho physiologically sensitive period for programming future physiology and behavior. It wasn't until births began taking place in hospitals that mothers and newborns were separated, completely or by clothing, after birth.

There is good evidence that normal term newborns who are placed skin to skin with their mothers immediately after birth make the transition from fetal to newborn life with greater respiratory, temperature, and glucose stability and significantly less crying indicating decreased stress. Mothers who hold their newborns skin to skin after birth have increased maternal behaviors, show more confidence in caring for their babies and breastfeed for longer durations. Being skin to skin protects your newborn from the well documented negative effects of separation, supports optimal brain development and facilitates attachment, which promotes your infant's self-regulation over time. Normal babies are born with the instinctive skill and motivation to breastfeed and are able to find the breast and self-attach without assistance when skin to skin. When your newborn is placed skin to skin with you, nine observable behaviors can be seen that lead to the first breastfeeding, usually within the first hour after birth (Moore E.R., 2012).

Skin to skin not only applies to moms, there are benefits for dads and partners being skin to skin with a baby as well. Your partner can be especially helpful with skin to skin contact in cases of a cesarean where mom may not be able to hold their baby immediately or with multiples. This contact with your partner will help regulate your baby's temperature, keep them calm, and promote bonding. Skin to skin contact extends through the first few weeks and is advised even after you are home with your baby.

The evidence to support immediate skin to skin contact is becoming more available all over the world. A study in Russia found that skin to skin contact positively influenced mother-infant interaction one year later when compared with routines involving separation of mother and infant (Bystrova, 2009). A study in India found that skin to skin contact improved physical growth of low birth weight infants (Gathwala G., 2010). There is overwhelming evidence that supports the benefits of skin to skin contact to both parents and babies. Immediate skin to skin contact is critical.

Vitamin K

Babies naturally have low levels of vitamin K at birth. A shot of vitamin K reduces the chance of vitamin K deficiency bleeding which happens in a small number of babies, and can be fatal. There are three types of this complication classified by when it occurs. Early, within 24 hours, and classical, within the first week, affects between 1 in 60 to 1 in 250 newborns. Late, within the first six months, is more rare and affects between 1 in 14,000 to 1 in 250,000 infants. Infants who do not receive a vitamin K shot at birth are 81 times more likely to develop vitamin K deficiency bleeding (Centers for Disease Control and Prevention, 2014).

The good news is that vitamin K deficiency bleeding can be prevented with a shot of vitamin K. The shot is given in your baby's thigh and it is stored in the muscle and released over a period of time and is designed to provide vitamin K until your baby is producing enough on their own. Since the early 1960s this has become standard procedure at all hospitals and birth centers. The shot is usually done within the first six hours after birth. This is a procedure that can be done while your baby is on your chest.

One risk factor for vitamin K deficiency is exclusively breastfeeding. Babies who are fed formula have higher levels of Vitamin K. By about six months of age your baby will be producing a sufficient amount of vitamin K on their own.

The only reason to include vitamin K in your birth plan is if you are opting out of the procedure or delaying it. If you have any questions or concerns about the safety of the shot, discuss them with your care provider to make sure you are making the best decision for your baby.

For more information on vitamin K you can listen to episode 47 of the Pregnancy Podcast at PregnancyPodcast.com/episode47.

Erythromycin

Ophthalmia neonatorum (ON) is conjunctivitis, or pink eye, that is contracted at birth. This eye infection is primarily caused by two sexually transmitted infections, gonorrhea and chlamydia. If you have either of these infections it can infect your newborn with ON. Untreated, ON can cause permanent eye damage or blindness. Many women who are infected with gonorrhea or chlamydia do not show any signs of infection and it has become standard practice to test for this in pregnancy.

It has become routine procedure for erythromycin eye ointment to be placed on your baby's eyes within 24 hours after birth. In the United States many states require by law that newborns are given erythromycin. The eye ointment can make your baby's vision temporarily blurry and it will wear away within 24 hours.

Some parents choose to opt out of this procedure, if their state allows it, if the mother does not have gonorrhea or chlamydia, and if they are in a monogamous relationship with one partner who is not infected. If you think erythromycin is a procedure you would like to decline, talk to your care provider about all of the risks, and find out if declining it is an option for you, and whether it is mandated by your state.

For more information on erythromycin you can listen to episode 47 of the Pregnancy Podcast at PregnancyPodcast.com/episode47.

Part Three: Guide to Writing Your Birth Plan

Chapter 14: Step-by-step Guide

You start creating your birth plan the minute you start educating yourself about labor and birth. This is going to be a work in progress throughout your pregnancy and it may change as you go. To be on the safe side you are going to want to have your birth plan done by week 36, but you can always make changes to it. You may find that you are even changing your priorities during labor depending on how your birth unfolds. You will want a few printed copies packed in your birth center or hospital bag, or on hand for a home birth. More importantly, you, your partner, your doula, and your care provider need to know what is included in your birth plan so you can all work together to create the birth experience you have been planning for.

By this point you are really knowledgeable about everything that can happen during birth and should have a solid idea of how you envision your birth. As you have been reading this book you have already completed some of the steps in the checklist below. Below is a step-by-step guide to creating your birth plan.

1. Get educated. Education about birth comes from reading resources like this book, listening to the Pregnancy Podcast, doing your own online research, and talking to your care provider.

2. Decide what is important and make a list. Get out a pen and paper, or a new Word document and start writing down the things that are important to you and that you know you want to include in your plan.

3. Find out what the policies are of your care provider or venue and make note as to whether they are in line with your wishes.

4. Create your first draft. Once you know the policies and routine procedures that will affect you birth you can compare these to your list and see what is in sync and what isn't. If you have a preference that is in line with your care provider's routine practice you may be able to take it out of your birth plan. On the other hand, if you wish to do something that is outside of your care provider's routine practice you will want to leave it in your birth plan to make sure they know your preference. You can use the template in the next section as a guide.

5. Check for conflicts. Read through your draft birth plan and see if everything makes sense and if there are any conflicts. For example,

you may not be able to avoid IV fluids if you are choosing to have your labor induced with Pitocin. Make sure everything in your plan works together.

6. Discuss it with your partner. Have your partner take a look at it and ask them if it makes sense or if you are leaving anything out.

7. Discuss it with your care provider. You will be working with your doctor or midwife throughout your entire pregnancy. If you aren't 100% clear on anything about your birth, now is the time to bring it up. Make sure your care provider is clear on what you want and that they are supportive of your wishes.

8. Final edits, make it short. Read through your birth plan and cut it down to one page. You could go longer if you feel it is really necessary but the shorter the better. One page is ideal. Ask yourself whether every item must be included. If a routine procedure is in line with what you want you can probably take it out of your birth plan. Focus on the things that are really important to you. Once you have a concise plan that you are happy with print it out.

9. Know it inside and out. You need to know exactly what is in your birth plan and be confident in your decisions so you know how you expect things to go down during your birth. This is also true for your partner. They need to know your birth plan well so in the event they need to speak up and advocate for you they can. If you are working with a doula also make sure they have a copy and will be supportive of your choices and know exactly what is important to you.

10. Pack it in your hospital or birth center bag, or have it on hand for your home birth. You should have a few copies printed out and make sure that the when you first see a nurse, midwife, or doctor they know that you have a birth plan so they can plan your care accordingly.

Part Four: Template and Samples

The birth plan template is available as a PDF at:
PregnancyPodcast.com/bptemplate
To access the document you will need to enter the password: YBP09temp26
This template includes everything you could include in your birth plan for a variety of births. Please feel free to delete, add, and customize it as you see fit.

Birth Plan Template

Dear [Hospital Staff, Birth Center Staff, Your Doctor, Your Midwife, Your Doula],

I appreciate you being here to support me through the birth of my first child!
I am so thankful to have your support during the birth of my baby!

I have spent a lot of time researching the evidence for all of the decisions listed here, and I feel confident in the choices I have made.
I have put a lot of time and energy into researching all of the evidence for my choices, and I feel confident in my birth wishes.

I thank you for respecting my wishes, especially if they fall outside of the usual procedure.
Thank you for supporting my wishes, especially if they do not align with your routine procedures.

I have been preparing and planning for a VBAC and am confident in this choice. I would like to exhaust all options for a successful vaginal birth before resorting to a C-section.

I have been preparing and planning for a natural birth and would like to avoid all interventions.
I would like to be paired up with a nurse who supports natural childbirth.

I have been preparing and planning for a [home/birth center] birth and would like to avoid a transfer to a hospital providing myself and my baby are doing well.

I have been preparing and planning for a water birth I would like to labor in water.
I would like to give birth to my baby [in water/on dry land].

I have been preparing for a [home/birth center] birth. If I am in the hospital, it is because I required some intervention that was unavailable.

I have been preparing and planning for a cesarean section

Environment:

The following people will be present during my labor and birth: [partner, doula, sister, brother, best friend, mother, father, photographer, etc.]
I value my privacy and would like to limit the number of staff members present to as few as possible.

It is my intent to give birth in a calm and relaxed environment.
I would like to keep the environment dimly lit, please dim or turn off any lighting when not needed.
I would like to keep my environment as quiet as possible with soft voices and minimal sound.
I would like to play [music, meditations, etc.] during my labor.
I would like to use essential oils and aromatherapy during my labor.

In labor:

I am not intent on delivering in a particular position or in a particular place. Please encourage me to try different things to see what works best.
It is my preference to labor in an upright position as much as possible, please encourage me to stay off of my back.
It is my preference to be as mobile as possible during my labor, please encourage me to try different positions.
I would like to include a [birthing ball, squatting bar, a birthing stool, etc.] for my labor. Please encourage me to utilize different props.

I prefer to avoid routine procedures (continuous EFM, IV, epidural, Pitocin augmentation, etc.) unless clearly necessary for a safe birth.
I am prepared to be flexible on the use of interventions if a medical necessity arises.
Barring a major medical emergency, I ask that you please discuss with me any and all interventions, allowing me the opportunity to give informed consent to any procedure you suggest.

I am comfortable inducing labor anytime after [41/42] weeks via [any method you feel is appropriate, sweeping the membranes, synthetic prostaglandins—misoprostol or dinoprostone, a mechanical dilator—balloon or laminaria, or rupturing the membranes].
I prefer to avoid inducing labor via [any method, sweeping the membranes, synthetic prostaglandins—misoprostol or dinoprostone, a mechanical dilator—balloon or laminaria, or rupturing the membranes].

I prefer to wait until at least [41/42] weeks to induce labor.

I am planning to be monitored using [external/internal] continuous electronic fetal monitoring.
I would like any monitoring to be intermittent.
I would like to have intermittent monitoring done via auscultation.
I would like to avoid internal continuous monitoring.
I would like to be monitored with a telemetry unit if possible to allow for the most mobility.

I am comfortable being given IV fluids throughout my labor.
I prefer to avoid IV fluids throughout my labor if possible.
I prefer a hep-lock in place of IV fluids.
In the event IV fluids are administered, it is important to me that you take the 24-hour birth weight of our baby into consideration to measure their weight gain.

I am group B strep positive and am planning on being given antibiotics during my labor. [Please note that I am allergic to penicillin.]

I am planning to have an [epidural/spinal] to assist with managing my contractions.
I would like [to have an epidural/spinal as soon as possible, or to hold off on having an epidural/spinal until I am at least 4/5/6/7 centimeters.]
I would like to keep the medication in my epidural to a minimum so that I may maintain some feeling.
I would like to use patient controlled medication so that I may be in control of the dosage.
Please do not offer an epidural or any medication, unless I request it.

I am comfortable using Pitocin to augment my labor.
I prefer not use Pitocin or any other method of augmentation.

Please do not perform an episiotomy unless necessary to prevent a second/third/fourth degree tear, or if medically necessary for an assisted delivery.
I would like to avoid an episiotomy if possible.
Please use [perineal massage, a warm compress, lubricant, or guided pushing] to prevent tearing or an episiotomy.
In the event an episiotomy becomes necessary it is my preference to use a [midline/median] incision.

If an assisted delivery becomes necessary I prefer to use [a ventouse suction cup/forceps].

I would like to avoid an assisted delivery.

In the event a hospital transfer is necessary for a non-emergency reason, I would like to be transferred to [hospital name].

Please lower the screen just before delivery so I may see the birth of my baby.

My partner would like to catch our baby when [he/she/they] are born.

It is important to me to utilize all other resources before a cesarean section.
In the event all other options are exhausted and a cesarean becomes necessary, I would like my partner present for the procedure.
In the event of a cesarean I would like the incision to be stitched up in two layers.

After the birth:

Please delay clamping of my baby's umbilical cord [for a minimum of 1/3/10 minutes/until it stops pulsating].
Please do not cut my baby's umbilical cord, I am planning a lotus birth.
My partner would like the opportunity to cut our baby's umbilical cord.

Please allow for the placenta to be delivered naturally and I request that you do not rush this process.
I am comfortable with active management for the third stage of labor.
I request no routine uterotonics to assist in the delivery of the placenta.
Please do not use [Pitocin/Carbetocin/Syntometrine/Cytotec].
Please do not apply controlled traction on the umbilical cord.

I am planning to keep and take my placenta home with me.
Someone will be picking up my placenta to prepare it for encapsulation.

I will be banking my baby's cord blood, after a delay of [1/2/3/10] minutes.

For my baby:

It is very important to me to be skin to skin with my baby immediately following birth.
Please perform any procedures or evaluations of my baby while they are on my chest.
In the event I am unable to be skin to skin with my baby immediately after birth please put my baby skin to skin with my partner.

I would like to breastfeed my baby as soon as possible after birth.

Please do not give my baby any infant formula.
In the event I decide to supplement with formula I have a specific brand I would like to use with me.

Please do not give my baby a pacifier.

I do not wish to give my baby a vitamin K shot.
Please delay the shot of vitamin K for 3/4/5/6+ hours.

I do not wish to give my baby erythromycin.
Please delay erythromycin for 1/12/24+ hours.
I [tested positive for gonorrhea/chlamydia and] would like erythromycin administered to my baby.

Thank you!
Thank you for taking good care of my baby and me!
I appreciate your support and care!

Your name

Sample Home Birth Plan

Dear Sara Smith, CNM,

I appreciate you being here to support me through the birth of my daughter! I have spent a lot of time researching the evidence for all of the decisions listed here, and I feel confident in the choices I have made. I have been preparing and planning for a home birth and would like to avoid a transfer to a hospital providing my baby and myself are doing well.

Environment:
The following people will be present during my labor and birth: my partner, Shannon, and my doula Caitlin. It is my intent to give birth in a calm and relaxed environment with dim lighting and soft voices.

In labor:
It is my preference to labor in an upright position as much as possible, please encourage me to stay off of my back. I would like to include a birthing ball and a birthing stool for my labor. Please use perineal massage, a warm compress, lubricant, and guided pushing to prevent tearing. My partner would like to catch our baby when she is born.

After the birth:
I would like to delay clamping of my baby's umbilical cord until it stops pulsating.
Please allow for the placenta to be delivered naturally and I request that you do not rush this process. Julia, from Julia's Birth Care, will be picking up my placenta to prepare it for encapsulation.

For my baby:
It is very important to me to be skin to skin with my baby immediately following birth and I would like to breastfeed my baby as soon as possible. I appreciate you giving my partner and I as much alone time with our new baby as possible.

Thank you for taking good care of my baby and me!

Joan

Sample Birth Center Birth Plan

Dear Birth Center Staff,

I am so thankful to have your support during the birth of my baby! I have put a lot of time and energy into researching all of the evidence for my choices, and I feel confident in my birth wishes. I have been preparing for a birth center birth and would like to avoid a transfer to a hospital providing my baby and myself are doing well. I thank you for respecting my wishes.

Environment:
My partner, Robert, and best friend and photographer, Alli, will be present during my labor and birth. It is my intent to give birth in a calm and relaxed environment. I would like to keep the environment dimly lit, with soft voices and minimal sound.

In labor:
It is my preference to labor in an upright position, please encourage me to stay off of my back. I would like to include a birthing ball for my labor.
To help prevent tearing, please use perineal massage, a warm compress, lubricant, and guided pushing.
My partner, Robert, would like to catch our baby when he is born.
In the event a hospital transfer is necessary for a non-emergency reason, I would like to be transferred to Sharp Hospital. Please coordinate my care with Dr. William Erickson.

After the birth:
Please delay clamping of my baby's umbilical cord for 10 minutes or until it stops pulsating.
Please allow for the placenta to be delivered naturally and I request that you do not rush this process.
Mary, from Living Tree Birth Services, will be picking up my placenta.

For my baby:
It is very important to me to be skin to skin with my baby immediately following birth. Please perform any procedures or evaluations of my baby while they are on my chest.
I would like to breastfeed my baby as soon as possible after birth.
Please delay the shot of vitamin K and erythromycin eye ointment for 6 hours.

I appreciate your support and care!

Jean

Sample Hospital Birth Plan – Plan B to Home or Birth Center

Dear Hospital Staff,

I am so thankful to have your support during the birth of my baby! I would like to be paired up with a nurse who supports natural childbirth. I have been preparing for a home birth, and if I am in the hospital, it is because I required some intervention that was unavailable.

Environment:
The following people will be present during my labor and birth: my partner, Steven, my doula, Evelyn, and my mother, Sarah.
It is my intent to give birth in a calm and relaxed environment. I would like to keep the environment dimly lit, please dim or turn off any lighting when not needed.

In labor:
I would like to include a squatting bar and a birthing stool for my labor.
I prefer to avoid routine procedures (continuous EFM, IV, epidural, Pitocin augmentation, etc.) unless clearly necessary for a safe birth. I am prepared to be flexible on the use of interventions if a medical necessity arises. Barring a major medical emergency, I ask that you please discuss with me any and all interventions, allowing me the opportunity to give informed consent to any procedure you suggest.
If continuous monitoring becomes necessary, I would like to be monitored with a telemetry unit if possible.
In the event IV fluids are administered, it is important to me that you take the 24-hour birth weight of our baby into consideration to measure their weight gain.
Please do not perform an episiotomy, unless necessary to prevent a third or fourth degree tear, or if medically necessary for an assisted delivery. If an assisted delivery becomes necessary I prefer to use a ventouse suction cup.
In the event all other options are exhausted and a cesarean becomes necessary, I would like my partner present for the procedure.

After the birth:
Please delay clamping of my baby's umbilical cord for a minimum of 3 minutes.
Please allow for the placenta to be delivered naturally and I request that you do not rush this process. If active management becomes necessary, please do not use Cytotec.

For my baby:

It is very important to me to be skin to skin with my baby immediately following birth. Please perform any procedures or evaluations of my baby while they are on my chest. In the event I am unable to be skin to skin with my baby immediately after birth please put my baby skin to skin with my partner.

I would like to breastfeed my baby as soon as possible after birth. Please do not give my baby any infant formula or a pacifier.

I appreciate your support and care!

Flora

Sample Hospital Birth Plan – Without Interventions

Dear Hospital Staff,

I appreciate you being here to support me through the birth of my daughter! I have spent a lot of time researching the evidence for all of the decisions listed here, and I feel confident in the choices I have made. I have been preparing and planning for a natural birth and would like to avoid all interventions. Please pair me up with a nurse who supports natural childbirth.

Environment:
My husband John, and sister Kate will be present during my labor and birth. I value my privacy and would like to limit the number of staff members present to as few as possible.
It is my intent to give birth in a calm and relaxed environment. Please dim or turn off any lighting when not needed. I would like to play music and incorporate aromatherapy during my labor.

In labor:
It is my preference to labor in an upright position as much as possible. Please encourage me to stay off of my back and try different positions.
I prefer to avoid routine procedures (continuous EFM, IV, epidural, Pitocin augmentation, etc.) unless clearly necessary for a safe birth. Barring a major medical emergency, I ask that you please discuss with me any and all interventions, allowing me the opportunity to give informed consent to any procedure you suggest.
Please do not offer an epidural or any medication, unless I request it.
To help prevent tearing, please use perineal massage, a warm compress, lubricant, or guided pushing.
It is important to me to utilize all other resources before a cesarean section. In the event all other options are exhausted and a cesarean becomes necessary, I would like my husband present for the procedure, and for you to lower the screen so I may see my daughter when she is born.

After the birth:
Please delay clamping of my baby's umbilical cord until it stops pulsating. My husband would like the opportunity to cut our baby's umbilical cord.
Please allow for the placenta to be delivered naturally and I request that you do not rush this process.

For my baby:
It is very important to me to be skin to skin with my baby immediately following birth. Please perform any procedures or evaluations of my baby while they are on my chest.

I would like to breastfeed as soon as possible after birth. In the event I decide to supplement with formula I have a specific brand I would like to use with me.

Please delay the shot of vitamin K and erythromycin eye ointment for 6 hours.

Thank you for taking good care of my baby and me!

Kara

Sample Hospital Birth Plan – With Interventions

Dear Hospital Staff,

I appreciate you being here to support me through the birth of my first child! I have spent a lot of time researching the evidence for all of the decisions listed here, and I feel confident in the choices I have made. Thank you for supporting my wishes.

Environment:
My partner, Mike, will be present during my labor and birth. It is my intent to give birth in a calm and relaxed environment. Please dim or turn off any lighting when not needed and use soft voices and minimal sound.

In labor:
It is my preference to labor in an upright position as much as possible, please encourage me to stay off of my back.
I am prepared to be flexible on the use of interventions if a medical necessity arises.
I am comfortable inducing labor anytime after 42 weeks via any method you feel is appropriate.
I am comfortable being given IV fluids throughout my labor.
I would like to have an epidural as soon as possible and I am comfortable using Pitocin to augment my labor.
In the event all other options are exhausted and a cesarean becomes necessary, I would like my partner present for the procedure.

After the birth:
Please delay clamping of my baby's umbilical cord for a minimum of 3 minutes.
I am comfortable with active management for the third stage of labor.

For my baby:
It is very important to me to be skin to skin with my baby immediately following birth and in the event I am unable to be skin to skin with my baby immediately after birth please put my baby skin to skin with my partner.
I would like to breastfeed my baby as soon as possible after birth.

Thank you for taking good care of my baby and me!

Liz

Sample Cesarean Section Birth Plan

Dear Hospital Staff,

I am so thankful to have your support during the birth of my baby! I have spent a lot of time researching the evidence for all of the decisions listed here, and I feel confident in the choices I have made. Thank you for supporting my wishes, especially if they do not align with your routine procedures. I have been preparing and planning for a cesarean section

Environment:
My partner, Brian, will be present during my birth.
It is my intent to give birth in a calm and relaxed environment. Please use low voices during the procedure.

During birth:
Please lower the screen just before delivery so I may see the birth of my baby. We have chosen not to find out the sex of our baby and I would like my partner to announce the sex when he or she is born.

After the birth:
Please delay clamping of my baby's umbilical cord for a minimum of 3 minutes.

For my baby:
It is very important to me to be skin to skin with my baby immediately following birth. If possible, please perform any procedures or evaluations of my baby while they are on my chest. In the event I am unable to be skin to skin with my baby immediately after birth please put my baby skin to skin with my partner.
I would like to breastfeed my baby as soon as possible. In the event I decide to supplement with formula I have a specific brand I would like to use with me.
Please delay erythromycin for 24 hours.

Thank you for taking good care of my baby and me!

Melissa

Additional Resources

PregnancyPodcast.com
The home base where you can get access to all of the Pregnancy Podcast episodes and links to additional resources, research, and studies.

Pregnancy Podcast
A podcast dedicated to all things pregnancy, birth, and being a new parent. A new episode is released every Sunday about a specific topic on pregnancy, birth, and being a new parent. Every Wednesday Vanessa answers a question from a listener with a short Q&A episode. You can find the Pregnancy Podcast on iTunes, Stitcher, and Google Play or listen to episodes directly on the website at PregnancyPodcast.com.

Pregnancy Podcast Community on Facebook
Connect with other expecting parents and ask questions specifically to what you are going through during pregnancy and what you are planning for your birth.

40 Weeks
A short podcast episode for each week of pregnancy. Find out what is going on with your body, how your baby is growing, plus get a weekly tip for dad, all in less than five minutes. You can find the podcast on iTunes, Stitcher, and Google Play or listen to episodes directly on the website at PregnancyPodcast.com/week. You can sign up with your email address to get a link to each week in your inbox according to your due date.

Vanessa Merten
The author of Your Birth Plan and host of the Pregnancy Podcast is committed to helping expecting parents navigate pregnancy, birth, and being a new parent. As always you can contact Vanessa through the Pregnancy podcast website or send her an email at vanessa@pregnancypodcast.com

All About Breastfeeding
Lori Isenstadt is a powerhouse of knowledge when it comes to everything Breastfeeding. She has many certifications in the maternity field, has worked as a childbirth educator, postpartum and birth doula, she has written several books, and for the last 20 years has worked as an International Board Certified Lactation Consultant. She is a pro on all things breastfeeding, she runs a private practice where she helps moms and babies with breastfeeding, and is the proud host of the All About Breastfeeding Podcast at AllAboutBreastfeeding.biz

La Leche League

An international organization dedicated to helping mothers worldwide to breastfeed through mother-to-mother support, encouragement, information, and education, and to promote a better understanding of breastfeeding as an important element in the healthy development of the baby and mother. The Womanly Art of Breastfeeding is the best selling guide to everything you need to know on breastfeeding. This book covers everything from preparing during pregnancy to troubleshooting. For more about La Leche League you can visit LLLI.org

Works Cited

Alfirevic Z., D. D. (2013, May 31). *Comparing continuous electronic fetal monitoring in labour (cardiotocography, CTG) with intermittent listening (intermittent auscultation, IA)*. Retrieved from http://www.cochrane.org/CD006066/PREG_comparing-continuous-electronic-fetal-monitoring-in-labour-cardiotocography-ctg-with-intermittent-listening-intermittent-auscultation-ia

American Academy of Pediatrics. (2007, January). *Cord Blood Banking for Potential Future Transplantation*. Retrieved from American Academy of Pediatrics: http://pediatrics.aappublications.org/content/119/1/165

American Academy of Pediatrics. (2014, April). *Immersion in Water During Labor and Delivery*. Retrieved from http://pediatrics.aappublications.org/content/133/4/758

American Academy of Pediatrics. (2011). *SIDS and Other Sleep-Related Infant Deaths: Expansion of Recommendations for a Safe Infant Sleeping Environment.* Retrieved from http://pediatrics.aappublications.org/content/early/2011/10/12/peds.2011-2284

American College of Nurse Midwives. (2014, April). *Hydrotherapy During Labor and Birth*. Retrieved from http://www.midwife.org/acnm/files/ccLibraryFiles/Filename/000000004048/Hydrotherapy-During-Labor-and-Birth-April-2014.pdf

American Congress of Obstetricians and Gynecologists & The American Academy of Pediatrics. (2014, April). *Immersion in Water During Labor and Delivery*. Retrieved from http://www.acog.org/Resources-And-Publications/Committee-Opinions/Committee-on-Obstetric-Practice/Immersion-in-Water-During-Labor-and-Delivery

American Congress of Obstetricians and Gynecologists Committee on Obstetric Practice. (2012, December). *Timing of Umbilical Cord Clamping After Birth*. Retrieved from http://www.acog.org/Resources-And-Publications/Committee-Opinions/Committee-on-Obstetric-Practice/Timing-of-Umbilical-Cord-Clamping-After-Birth

American Congress of Obstetricians and Gynecologists. (2011). *Planned Home Birth Committee Opinion*. Retrieved from http://www.acog.org/Resources-And-Publications/Committee-Opinions/Committee-on-Obstetric-Practice/Planned-Home-Birth

American Congress of Obstetricians and Gynecologists. (2015, December). *Umbilical Cord Blood Banking*. Retrieved from http://www.acog.org/Resources-And-Publications/Committee-Opinions/Committee-on-Genetics/Umbilical-Cord-Blood-Banking

American Congress of Obstetricians and Gynecologists. (2010, August). *Vaginal Birth After Previous Cesarean Delivery*. Retrieved from http://www.acog.org/Resources-And-Publications/Practice-Bulletins/Committee-on-Practice-Bulletins-Obstetrics/Vaginal-Birth-After-Previous-Cesarean-Delivery

American Medical Association. (2008, June). *Opinion 2.165 - Umbilical Cord Blood Banking*. Retrieved from http://www.ama-assn.org/ama/pub/physician-resources/medical-ethics/code-medical-ethics/opinion2165.page?

Anim-Somuah M., S. R. (2011, December 7). *Epidurals for pain relief in labour*. Retrieved from http://www.cochrane.org/CD000331/PREG_epidurals-for-pain-relief-in-labour

Australian Institute of Health and Welfare. (2013). *Australia's Mothers and Babies 2013*. Retrieved from http://www.aihw.gov.au/WorkArea/DownloadAsset.aspx?id=60129554140

Begley CM, G. G. (2015, March 2). *Delivering the placenta with active, expectant or mixed management in the third stage of labour*. Retrieved from http://www.cochrane.org/CD007412/PREG_delivering-the-placenta-with-active-expectant-or-mixed-management-in-the-third-stage-of-labour

Blondel B., A. S.-R.-A.-M., & Committee, &. E.-P. (2016, April 5). *Variations in rates of severe perineal tears and episiotomies in 20 European countries: a study based on routine national data in Euro-Peristat Project*. Retrieved from http://www.ncbi.nlm.nih.gov/pubmed/26958827

Bodner-Adler B., B. K. (2003, April). *Management of the perineum during forceps delivery. Association of episiotomy with the frequency and severity of perineal trauma in women undergoing forceps delivery*. Retrieved from http://www.ncbi.nlm.nih.gov/pubmed/12746986

Bujold E., B. C. (2002, June). *The impact of a single-layer or double-layer closure on uterine rupture*. Retrieved from http://www.ncbi.nlm.nih.gov/pubmed/12066117

Bujold E., G. M. (2010, July). *The role of uterine closure in the risk of uterine rupture.* Retrieved from http://www.ncbi.nlm.nih.gov/pubmed/20567166

Bystrova, K. I.-A.-M. (2009, May 28). *Early Contact versus Separation: Effects on Mother–Infant Interaction One Year Later.* Retrieved from http://onlinelibrary.wiley.com/doi/10.1111/j.1523-536X.2009.00307.x/abstract

Caughey A.B., C. A. (2014, March 1). *Obstetric Care Consensus.* Retrieved from The American Congress of Obtetricians and Gynecologists: http://www.acog.org/Resources-And-Publications/Obstetric-Care-Consensus-Series/Safe-Prevention-of-the-Primary-Cesarean-Delivery

Centers for Disease Control and Prevention. (2014, March 31). *Facts about Vitamin K Deficiency Bleeding.* Retrieved from http://www.cdc.gov/ncbddd/vitamink/facts.html#ref

Cluett, E. &. (2009, April 15). *Immersion in water in labour and birth.* Retrieved from http://onlinelibrary.wiley.com/doi/10.1002/14651858.CD000111.pub3/abstract;jsessionid=90BC5178CDECB0FA280C6CCEE44A73E0.f04t01

Coyle C., H. K. (2014). *Placentophagy: therapeutic miracle or myth?* Retrieved from https://www.researchgate.net/publication/277779644_Placentophagy_Therapeutic_miracle_or_myth

Dekker. (2013, January 31). *National Birth Center Study II.* Retrieved from http://www.birthcenters.org/?page=NBCSII

Department of Reproductive Health and Research World Health Organization. (2015). *WHO Statement on Caesarean Section Rates.* Retrieved from World Health Organization: http://apps.who.int/iris/bitstream/10665/161442/1/WHO_RHR_15.02_eng.pdf?ua=1

Devane D., L. J. (2012, February 15). *Comparing electronic monitoring of the baby's heartbeat on a woman's admission in labour using cardiotocography (CTG) with intermittent monitoring.* Retrieved from http://onlinelibrary.wiley.com/doi/10.1002/14651858.CD005122.pub4/abstract;jsessionid=2F09C7BEF69F7F76C71631054365E120.f03t04

Durnwald C., M. B. (2003, October). *Uterine rupture, perioperative and perinatal morbidity after single-layer and double-layer closure at cesarean delivery.* Retrieved from http://www.ncbi.nlm.nih.gov/pubmed/14586327

French C.A., C. X. (2016, April 27). *Labor Epidural Analgesia and Breastfeeding: A Systematic Review*. Retrieved from http://www.ncbi.nlm.nih.gov/pubmed/27121239

Gaskin, I. M. (2013, September). *Cytotec and the FDA*. Retrieved from Midwifery Today Web Site: https://www.midwiferytoday.com/articles/cytotec_fda.asp

Gaskin, I. M. (n.d.). *Reprint of Email From Ina May Gaskin*. Retrieved June 10, 2016, from College of Midwives: http://www.collegeofmidwives.org/collegeofmidwives.org/news01/VBAC%20gaskin01a.htm

Gathwala G., S. B. (2010, October). *Effect of Kangaroo Mother Care on physical growth, breastfeeding and its acceptability*. Retrieved from http://tdo.sagepub.com/content/40/4/199.abstract?ct=ct#cited-by

Gizzo S., D. G. (2014, May 15). *Women's Choice of Positions during Labour: Return to the Past or a Modern Way to Give Birth? A Cohort Study in Italy*. (University of Padua Department of Woman and Child Health, Producer) Retrieved from http://www.hindawi.com/journals/bmri/2014/638093/

Grivell R.M., A. Z. (2015, September 12). *Cardiotocography (a form of electronic fetal monitoring) for assessing a baby's well-being in the womb during pregnancy*. Retrieved from http://www.cochrane.org/CD007863/PREG_cardiotocography-form-electronic-fetal-monitoring-assessing-babys-well-being-womb-during-pregnancy

Gupta J.K., H. G. (2012, May 16). *Position in the second stage of labour for women without epidural anaesthesia*. Retrieved from http://www.cochrane.org/CD002006/PREG_position-in-the-second-stage-of-labour-for-women-without-epidural-anaesthesia

Gyamfi C., J. G. (2006, October 19). *Single- versus double-layer uterine incision closure and uterine rupture*. Retrieved from http://www.ncbi.nlm.nih.gov/pubmed/17118738

Hanson L., V. L. (2014, April 22). *Feasibility of oral prenatal probiotics against maternal group B Streptococcus vaginal and rectal colonization*. Retrieved from http://www.ncbi.nlm.nih.gov/pubmed/24754328

Hart, G. (2010). *Midwifery Today Responds to Study Questioning Homebirth Safety*. Retrieved from https://www.midwiferytoday.com/articles/ajog_response.asp

Hartmann K., V. M. (2005, May 4). *Outcomes of Routine Episiotomy A Systematic Review*. Retrieved from http://jama.jamanetwork.com/article.aspx?articleid=200799

Hodnett E.D., G. S. (2012, October 17). *Continuous support for women during childbirth*. Retrieved from http://www.ncbi.nlm.nih.gov/pubmed/23076901

Hofmeyr GJ, M. N. (2015, January 29). *Controlled cord traction for the third stage of labour*. Retrieved from http://onlinelibrary.wiley.com/doi/10.1002/14651858.CD008020.pub2/abstract

Humphries, G. (2014, January). *The Suture Debate*. Retrieved from International Cesarean Awareness Network: http://www.ican-online.org/wp-content/uploads/2014/06/The-Suture-Debate.pdf

Institute for Quality and Efficiency in Health Care. (2012, July 19). *Pregnancy and birth: Epidurals and painkillers for labor pain relief*. Retrieved from http://www.ncbi.nlm.nih.gov/pubmedhealth/PMH0072751/

International Journal of Women's Health. (2015). *Table 2*. Retrieved from http://www.ncbi.nlm.nih.gov/pmc/articles/PMC4399594/table/t2-ijwh-7-361/

Jonge A., G. C. (2014, September 10). *Perinatal mortality and morbidity up to 28 days after birth among 743 070 low-risk planned home and hospital births: a cohort study based on three merged national perinatal databases*. Retrieved from http://onlinelibrary.wiley.com/doi/10.1111/1471-0528.13084/full

Lappen J.R., &. H. (2015). *Outcomes of Term Induction in Trial of Labor After Cesarean Delivery: Analysis of a Modern Obstetric Cohort*. Retrieved from http://www.ncbi.nlm.nih.gov/m/pubmed/26241264/?i=29&from=/2396239/related

Lawrence A., L. L. (2013, August 20). *Maternal positions and mobility during first stage labour*. Retrieved from http://www.ncbi.nlm.nih.gov/pubmed/19370591

MacDorman M.F., M. T. (2014, March). *Trends in Out-of-Hospital Births in the United States, 1990–2012*. Retrieved from http://www.cdc.gov/nchs/data/databriefs/db144.htm#x2013;2012</a>

March of Dimes. (2011, June). *Oligohydramnios*. Retrieved from March of Dimes: http://www.marchofdimes.org/complications/oligohydramnios.aspx

McDonald S.J., M. P. (2013, July 11). *Effect of timing of umbilical cord clamping of term infants on mother and baby outcomes.* Retrieved from http://onlinelibrary.wiley.com/doi/10.1002/14651858.CD004074.pub3/abstract

McDonald SJ, A. J. (2004, January 26). *Prophylactic ergometrine-oxytocin versus oxytocin for the third stage of labour.* (C. D. Reviews, Producer) Retrieved from http://onlinelibrary.wiley.com/wol1/doi/10.1002/14651858.CD000201.pub2/full

Midwives Alliance North America. (n.d.). *State by State.* Retrieved June 16, 2016, from Midwives Alliance North America: http://mana.org/about-midwives/state-by-state

Midwives Association of British Columbia. (2010). *Facts and Figures.* Retrieved from Midwives Association of British Columbia: http://www.bcmidwives.com/midwifery-facts-and-figures

Molina G., W. T.-L. (2015, December 1). *Relationship Between Cesarean Delivery Rate and Maternal and Neonatal Mortality.* Retrieved from http://jama.jamanetwork.com/article.aspx?articleid=2473490

Mollamahmutoğlu L., M. O. (2012, March 1). *The effects of immersion in water on labor, birth and newborn and comparison with epidural analgesia and conventional vaginal delivery.* Retrieved from http://www.ncbi.nlm.nih.gov/pmc/articles/PMC3940223/

Moore E.R., A. G. (2012, May 16). *Early skin-to-skin contact for mothers and their healthy newborn infants.* Retrieved from http://www.ncbi.nlm.nih.gov/pmc/articles/PMC3979156/

Murray-Davis B., &. R. (2015, April). *Choosing Where to Give Birth: Results of the Ontario Choice of Birthplace Study.* Retrieved from https://www.bornontario.ca/assets/documents/provincialrounds/Choosing%20Where%20to%20Give%20Birth%20-%20April%202015.pdf

Noel-Weiss J., W. A. (2011, August 15). *An observational study of associations among maternal fluids during parturition, neonatal output, and breastfed newborn weight loss.* Retrieved from http://www.ncbi.nlm.nih.gov/pubmed/21843338

Office for National Statistics. (2014, November 17). *Births in England and Wales by Characteristics of Birth 2: 2013.* Retrieved from http://www.ons.gov.uk/peoplepopulationandcommunity/birthsdeathsandma

rriages/livebirths/bulletins/characteristicsofbirth2/2014-11-17#tab-Key-Findings

O'Connor N.R., T. K. (2009). *Pacifiers and Breastfeeding a Systematic Review.* Retrieved from
http://archpedi.jamanetwork.com/article.aspx?articleid=381289

O'Mahony F., H. G. (2010, October 4). *Choice of instruments for assisted vaginal delivery.* Retrieved from
http://onlinelibrary.wiley.com/doi/10.1002/14651858.CD005455.pub2/abstract

Osterman M.J.K., &. M. (2011, April 6). *Epidural and Spinal Anesthesia Use During Labor: 27-state Reporting Area, 2008.* Retrieved from Centers for Disease Control and Prevention:
http://www.cdc.gov/nchs/data/nvsr/nvsr59/nvsr59_05.pdf

Osterman, M. &. (2014, November 5). *Trends in Low-risk Cesarean Delivery in the United States, 1990–2013.* Retrieved from
http://www.cdc.gov/nchs/data/nvsr/nvsr63/nvsr63_06.pdf

Rönnqvist P.D., F.-B. U.-H. (2006). *Lactobacilli in the female genital tract in relation to other genital microbes and vaginal pH.* Retrieved from
http://www.ncbi.nlm.nih.gov/pubmed/16752267

Rabe H., D.-R. J. (2012, August 15). *Early cord clamping versus delayed cord clamping or cord milking for preterm babies.* Retrieved from
http://onlinelibrary.wiley.com/doi/10.1002/14651858.CD003248.pub3/abstract

Smaill F.M., &. G. (2014, October 28). *Routine antibiotics at cesarean section to reduce infection.* Retrieved from
http://onlinelibrary.wiley.com/doi/10.1002/14651858.CD007482.pub3/abstract;jsessionid=1AEDD978FD0148470D2DD3A43F2D4B39.f03t02

Sooklim R., T. J. (2007, October 29). *The outcomes of midline versus medio-lateral episiotomy.* Retrieved from
http://www.ncbi.nlm.nih.gov/pmc/articles/PMC2174441/

Stanford University. (2014, November). *Effects of Oral Probiotic Supplementation on Group B Strep (GBS) Rectovaginal Colonization in Pregnancy.* Retrieved from
https://clinicaltrials.gov/ct2/show/NCT01479478?term=probiotics+AND+group+b+strep&rank=1

Takahashi. (2013, March 1). *UNLV researchers author first-ever scholarly report on experiences of placenta-eating moms*. Retrieved from http://lasvegassun.com/news/2013/mar/01/unlv-researchers-author-first-ever-scholarly-repor/

Thöni A., M. K. (2010, June). *Water birthing: retrospective review of 2625 water births. Contamination of birth pool water and risk of microbial cross-infection*. Retrieved from http://www.ncbi.nlm.nih.gov/m/pubmed/20595945/?i=31&from=%22water%20birth%22

Tunçalp Ö, H. G. (2012, August 15). *Prostaglandins for preventing postpartum haemorrhage*. Retrieved from http://onlinelibrary.wiley.com/wol1/doi/10.1002/14651858.CD000494.pub4/full

U.S. Food and Drug Administration. (2015, July 10). *Misoprostol (Marketed as Cytotec) Information*. Retrieved from U.S. Food and Drug Administration Web Site: http://www.fda.gov/Drugs/DrugSafety/PostmarketDrugSafetyInformationforPatientsandProviders/ucm111315

Wang L., Z. J. (2015, June 11). *Efficacy and safety of misoprostol compared with the dinoprostone for labor induction at term: a meta-analysis*. Retrieved from http://www.ncbi.nlm.nih.gov/pubmed/26067262

Westhoff G, C. A. (2013, October 30). *Prophylactic oxytocin for the third stage of labour to prevent postpartum haemorrhage*. Retrieved from http://onlinelibrary.wiley.com/doi/10.1002/14651858.CD001808.pub2/full

World Health Organization. (2014). *Guideline: Delayed umbilical cord clamping for improved maternal and infant health and nutrition outcomes*. Retrieved from World Health Organization: http://apps.who.int/iris/bitstream/10665/148793/1/9789241508209_eng.pdf

Zielinski R., A. K. (2015, April 8). *Planned home birth: benefits, risks, and opportunities*. Retrieved from http://www.ncbi.nlm.nih.gov/pmc/articles/PMC4399594/#b4-ijwh-7-361

Made in the USA
Columbia, SC
01 April 2020

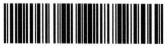